Maternal-Newborn Nursing Care: A Workbook

REVISED EDITION

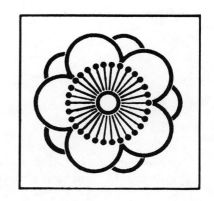

Maternal-Newborn Nursing Care: A Workbook

SALLY B. OLDS, R.N., M.S.N.
Coordinator Maternal-Child Nursing
Beth-El School of Nursing
Colorado Springs, Colorado

MARCIA L. LONDON, R.N., M.S.N., N.N.P.
Neonatal Nurse Practioner
Intensive Care Nursery
Memorial Hospital
Colorado Springs, Colorado

PATRICIA A. LADEWIG, R.N., M.S.N., N.P.
Assistant Professor
Loretto Heights College
Denver, Colorado
Doctoral Candidate
University of Denver

Addison-Wesley Publishing Company
Nursing Division, Menlo Park, California
Reading, Massachusetts • London • Amsterdam • Don Mills, Ontario • Sydney

Sponsoring Editor: Deborah Gale
Production Coordinator: Betty Duncan-Todd

Credits: p. 39: photo from Bloom, W., and Fawcett, D.W. 1975.
A textbook of histology. 10th ed. Philadelphia: W. B. Saunders Co.;
pp. 116-119, 163-166, 169: fetal monitoring paper courtesy of
Corometrics Medical Systems, Inc., Wallingford, Connecticut;
pp. 130-131: courtesy of Ross Laboratories, Columbus, Ohio 43216.

ISBN 0-201-12799-7

ABCEDFGHIJ-AL-89876543

The authors and publishers have exerted every effort to ensure that drug
selection and dosage set forth in this text are in accord with current
recommendations and practice at the time of publication. However, in
view of ongoing research, changes in government regulations and the
constant flow of information relating to drug therapy and drug reactions,
the reader is urged to check the package insert for each drug for any
change in indications of dosage and for added warnings and pre-
cautions. This is particularly important where the recommended agent is
a new and/or infrequently employed drug.

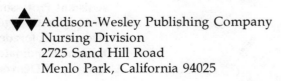 Addison-Wesley Publishing Company
Nursing Division
2725 Sand Hill Road
Menlo Park, California 94025

We dedicate this book to our families—
everchanging but always constant in their love.

Joe, Scott and Allison Olds

David, Craig and Matthew London

Tim, Ryan and Erik Ladewig

PREFACE

Maternity nurses are responsible for a complex, highly specialized body of knowledge that is designed to meet the needs of their clients—both normal and high-risk. In recent years that knowledge base has expanded rapidly. Related research, especially in the area of assessment of fetal status, has resulted in major improvements in the quality of care available for prenatal women and their unborn children.

Trends in maternity care are changing, too. The focus has returned to the family as co-participants in childbirth. Fathers are assuming an active role in labor and delivery. Consumer demand for a more meaningful childbirth experience has led to an increase in birthing room deliveries and even home births.

Nursing programs find themselves attempting to deal with this explosion of knowledge and with such complex bioethical issues as abortion, test-tube babies, fetal research, and euthanasia when there is barely enough time to present basic content.

We believe that *Maternal–Newborn Nursing Care: A Workbook* will aid maternity education by providing a concise, up-to-date review of essential theoretical content while emphasizing the application of the nursing process in a maternity setting.

Organization

Although the sequence varies somewhat, all major texts of maternity nursing include content related to the human reproductive system and to the antepartal, intrapartal, postpartal, and neonatal periods. *Maternal–Newborn Nursing Care: A Workbook* is designed to be used with most of the major maternity nursing texts, no matter what their organization.

Chapter 1 briefly introduces some pertinent concepts and then reviews examples of relevant statistical data. It concludes with a brief overview of selected theories related to the family.

Chapters 2 and 3 focus on the human reproductive system and the developing fetus. This review of anatomy and physiology helps students more clearly understand the changes that occur during the course of a pregnancy.

The physiologic and psychologic adaptations that occur during pregnancy are explored in Chapter 4. Chapter 5 focuses on the assessment and care of the normal antepartal family, and Chapter 6 considers the antepartal family that experiences complications.

Fetal assessment techniques have proliferated at an amazing rate, and Chapter 7 explores those that are fairly widely used at present.

Chapters 8 through 11 consider different aspects of the intrapartal period. These chapters first focus on the physiologic and psychologic changes that occur (Chapter 8), then consider the nursing assessment and care (Chapter 9). Chapter 10 provides a concise review of the methods of pain relief currently used in obstetrics, and Chapter 11 considers the high-risk labor and delivery client.

Chapter 12 includes the normal physiologic and psychologic responses of the puerperium and the appropriate nursing assessments, care, and evaluations. Chapter 13 considers postpartal complications.

In similar fashion, Chapter 14 considers the normal newborn, and Chapter 15 is devoted to the assessment and care of the high-risk neonate.

Pertinence for Clinical Practice

The nursing process forms the framework for nursing care today, and this workbook is designed to assist students in applying it. In keeping with current trends, this workbook emphasizes the development of pertinent assessment skills. This strong base in assessment can then be used to plan, analyze, implement, and evaluate nursing care.

Some of the items in *Maternal–Newborn Nursing Care: A Workbook* are related to essential factual material, and students may verify their answers in any of the major maternity nursing textbooks. However, some of the items require a degree of synthesis and application, and the answers may not readily be confirmed. In these instances we have established a dialogue with the student. The dialogues serve to assist the student with self-assessment because they provide possible solutions to items that require a nursing judgment. If students have failed to grasp certain content, they will find helpful recommendations about ways to restudy this material.

Because it is our belief that sound clinical judgment develops from both theoretical knowledge and practical experience, many of the items in this workbook are based on clinical situations. We hope in this way to assist students in the appropriate application of theory.

Pedagogic Aids

The subject areas included in this workbook were chosen to assist students in learning the most essential content of maternity nursing. Figures and tables have been included when they provide additional clarification or insight.

Items that are reviewed in a dialogue are marked with an asterisk and addressed at the end of Part I in each chapter.

Part II of each chapter is a Self-Assessment Guide composed of several multiple-choice items, and answers to all of these are provided. Students who have accurately completed the items in Part I should be able to successfully answer all the questions in Part II.

A Selected Bibliography at the end of each chapter provides direction and possible sources of information for students who seek clarification or additional information.

Applications

Maternal–Newborn Nursing Care: A Workbook is not a programmed text but an aid to students in learning maternity nursing content and in improving their skills in critical thinking. Because it is designed to supplement the major maternity nursing textbooks currently in use, it is of value to nursing students in all types of programs—baccalaureate, diploma, and associate degree. Nurses involved in refresher courses or entering this specialty area will also find this workbook essential. Practicing nurses may find it helpful, too, especially in the area of assessment.

Clarification of Terms

Although we recognize that male registered nurses are becoming more involved in the provision of maternity care, female nurses are still the major care providers. Therefore, whenever possible we have avoided assigning a sex to the nurse, but when this was not possible we have used the female pronoun.

By the same token, we appreciate the fact that the individual who is most significant to the pregnant woman may be her husband, the father of the child, a family member, or simply a good friend, male or female. Thus we have attempted to provide both traditional "husband-wife" situations and situations involving some other support person.

Acknowledgments

We wish to thank the nurse-educators and practicing maternity nurses who diligently reviewed this material and offered their suggestions and comments. In a book of this sort it is sometimes difficult to avoid regionalization and maintain a focus on the most pertinent material. Their input gave us a broader perspective and helped us when we occasionally suffered from "tunnel vision."

We wish especially to thank Pat Franklin Waldo and Deborah Gale, our editors, for their unfailing willingness to provide encouragement, humor, and support. We also thank Betty Duncan-Todd for her efforts in coordinating the revised edition of this workbook.

We wish to acknowledge the efforts of Beverly Watson and Jeannine Keyes in typing this manuscript. Their enthusiasm and competence were deeply appreciated.

Finally, we thank our families. During the course of our writing endeavors, they have grown and changed, but they have remained faithful allies and tremendous sources of love and support.

S.B.O.
M.L.L.
P.A.L.

CONTENTS

Maternal-Newborn Nursing Care: A Workbook

CHAPTER 1 MATERNITY NURSING: CHANGING PERSPECTIVES

INTRODUCTION

The broad scope of maternity nursing offers a variety of professional opportunities and greatly increases the quality of care available to childbearing families. Nurses today draw on their educational and professional expertise and also use family and statistical data in planning and providing care.

This chapter provides an introduction to the current roles of maternity nurses. It then focuses on pertinent statistical data. The latter portion of the chapter is designed to assist students in reading statistical tables and at the same time allow them to reflect briefly on the significance of the information provided in the tables.

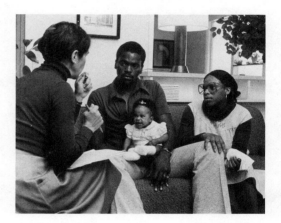

After reviewing statistical information, the chapter introduces selected theories related to family structure, development, and functioning. This introductory content is intended to provide a base for consideration of the care required by a family during its childbearing time.

PART I
GENERAL PRINCIPLES AND CONCEPTS

1. Maternity nurses function in a variety of roles in providing care to childbearing families. Define each of the following roles with emphasis on educational background and scope of function:

   a. Labor and delivery (clinic, postpartal, or newborn nursery) professional nurse

   b. Clinical nurse specialist

c. Nurse practitioner

d. Certified nurse-midwife (CNM)

2. What is meant by the term *lay midwife*?

3. Briefly discuss the concept of family-centered maternity care.

4. Identify five uses of statistical data in planning and providing nursing care.

a.

b.

c.

d.

e.

5. Define the following terms:

   a. Descriptive statistics

   b. Inferential statistics

   c. Birth rate

   d. Infant death rate

   e. Neonatal mortality

   f. Perinatal mortality

   g. Maternal mortality

4

Table 1-1. Estimated infant mortality per 1000 live births.

Age at death/ cause of death	November 1980		November 1979		January-November 1980		January-November 1979	
	Number	Rate	Number	Rate	Number	Rate	Number	Rate
Total, under 1 year	375	12.5	384	13.1	4,112	12.6	4,143	13.1
Under 28 days	251	8.5	260	8.8	2,772	8.5	2,804	8.8
28 days to 11 months	124	4.0	124	4.4	1,340	4.2	1,339	4.3
Certain gastrointestinal diseases	3	0.1	4	0.1	25	0.1	36	0.1
Pneumonia and influenza	4	0.1	11	0.4	94	0.3	102	0.3
Congenital anomalies	80	2.7	73	2.5	844	2.6	833	2.6
Disorders relating to short gestation and unspecified low birth weight	33	1.1	21	0.7	365	1.1	323	1.0
Birth trauma	7	0.2	10	0.3	79	0.2	102	0.3
Intrauterine hypoxia and birth asphyxia	16	0.5	22	0.7	141	0.4	155	0.5
Respiratory distress syndrome	35	1.2	48	1.6	456	1.4	505	1.6
Other conditions originating in the perinatal period	86	2.9	94	3.2	1,024	3.1	1,020	3.2
Sudden infant death syndrome	52	1.7	37	1.3	473	1.5	448	1.4
All other causes	59	1.9	64	2.2	621	1.9	619	2.0

From U.S. Department of Health and Human Services. March 18, 1981. Provisional Data from National Center for Health Statistics. *Monthly Vital Statistics Report*. Publication No.(PHS) 81-1120, p. 10. Vol. 29, No. 12.

6. Using Table 1-1, answer the following:

   a. What was the neonatal mortality for January-November 1980.* _____

   b. Of the selected causes of infant mortality that are listed, which had the highest rate in all cases?* _____

   c. Which of the causes had the lowest rate in November 1980?* _____

   d. What changes occurred in infant mortality from 1979 to 1980?* _____

   e. Briefly discuss the significance of the data in Table 1-1 in planning infant care.

*These questions are addressed at the end of Part I.

Table 1–2. Number and Percent Low Birth Weight, by Age of Mother and Race of Child, United States, 1980*

Age of mother and race of child	Percent low birth weight	Total	Birth weight[1]				
			Under 500	500–999	1000–1499	1500–1999	2000–2499
All races							
All ages	6.8	3,612,258	3,591	15,903	21.936	47,680	157,182
Under 15 years	14.6	10,169	32	162	150	326	812
15–19 years	9.4	552,161	663	3,516	4,955	10,285	32,401
20–24 years	6.9	1,226,200	1,223	5,263	7,325	16,100	54,689
25–29 years	5.8	1,108,291	980	4,212	5,569	12,219	41,282
30–34 years	5.9	550,354	515	2,075	2,879	6,252	20,580
35–39 years	7.0	140,793	153	571	854	2,068	6,166
40–44 years	8.3	23,090	24	100	187	403	1,192
45–49 years	9.2	1,200	1	4	17	27	60
White							
All ages	5.7	2,898,732	2,120	9,755	14,079	31,788	107,074
Under 15 years	11.2	4,171	10	46	50	117	241
15–19 years	7.7	388,058	329	1,897	2,830	5,901	18,869
20–24 years	5.7	982,526	694	3,142	4,607	10,633	36,924
25–29 years	5.0	933,159	643	2,837	3,881	8,843	30,572
30–34 years	5.1	459,151	334	1,394	2,018	4,566	15,142
35–39 years	6.2	113,124	95	371	566	1,413	4,486
40–44 years	7.4	17,652	14	65	117	295	806
45–49 years	7.7	891	1	3	10	20	34
All other							
All ages	11.5	713,526	1,471	6,148	7,857	15,892	50,108
Under 15 years	17.1	5,998	22	116	100	209	571
15–19 years	13.5	164,103	334	1,619	2,125	4,384	13,532
20–24 years	11.8	243,674	529	2,121	2,718	5,467	17,765
25–29 years	10.0	175,132	337	1,375	1,688	3,376	10,710
30–34 years	9.7	91,203	181	681	861	1,686	5,438
35–39 years	10.5	27,669	58	200	288	655	1,680
40–44 years	11.3	5,438	10	35	70	108	386
45–49 years	13.4	309	-	1	7	7	26
Black							
All ages	12.5	589,616	1,381	5,748	7,208	14,463	44,662
Under 15 years	17.2	5,793	22	115	96	203	558
15–19 years	14.0	150,353	323	1,568	2,038	4,182	12,828
20–24 years	12.6	209,596	508	2,010	2,547	5,085	16,245
25–29 years	11.2	135,680	311	1,248	1,534	2,977	9,112
30–34 years	11.1	64,369	156	603	687	1,390	4,307
35–39 years	11.7	19,631	53	173	242	537	1,287
40–44 years	12.2	3,990	8	31	61	83	302
45–49 years	15.8	204	-	-	3	6	23

*Based on 100% of births in selected states and on a 50% sample of births in all other states. Modified from National Center for Health Statistics: Advance report of final natality statistics, 1980. *Monthly vital statistics report.* Vol. 31, No. 8, Supp. DHHS Pub. No. (PHS) 83–1120. Public Health Service, Hyattsville, Md. November 1982.

[1]Equivalents of the gram weight in pounds and ounces are as follows:
Under 500 g = 1 lb, 1 oz or less
500–999 g = 1 lb, 2 oz–2 lb, 3 oz
1000–1499 g = 2 lb, 4 oz–3 lb, 4 oz
1500–1999 g = 3 lb, 5 oz–4 lb, 6 oz
2000–2499 g = 4 lb, 7 oz–5 lb, 8 oz

7. Using Table 1-2, answer the following:

   a. Define low birth weight.
   b. The highest percent of low birth weight babies occurred in mothers whose ages were _____, and whose race was _____.*
   c. In looking at the data under *all races*, the lowest percent of low birth weight babies were born to mothers of _____ years of age.*
   d. Compare the age range identified in the above question (7c) with data for *white* and *black* categories. Is the age range for lowest percent of low birth weight babies the same for white mothers? _____.*
      For black mothers? _____.*
   e. Briefly describe inferential considerations of the data provided in Table 1-2.

*These questions are addressed at the end of Part I.

Table 1-3. Infant Mortality Rates by Age: United States, 1950, 1960, 1965, and 1970–80*

Year	Under 1 year	Under 28 days	28 days–11 months
1980 (est.)	12.5	8.4	4.1
1979 (est.)	13.0	8.7	4.2
1978	13.8	9.5	4.3
1977	14.1	9.9	4.2
1976	15.2	10.9	4.3
1975	16.1	11.6	4.5
1974	16.7	12.3	4.4
1973	17.7	13.0	4.8
1972[1]	18.5	13.6	4.8
1971	19.1	14.2	4.9
1970	20.0	15.1	4.9
1965	24.7	17.7	7.0
1960	26.0	18.7	7.3
1950	29.2	20.5	8.7

*For 1979 and 1980, based on a 10% sample of deaths; for all other years, based on final data. Rates per 1000 live births. From National Center for Health Statistics: Advance report of final natality statistics. 1981. *Monthly vital statistics report*. Vol. 29. No. 13. Public Health Service, Hyattsville, Md. Sept. 17, 1981.

[1]Based on a 50% sample of deaths.

Table 1-4. U.S. Maternal Mortality Rate per 100,000 Live Births*

Year	Rate	Year	Rate
1980 (est.)	6.9	1969	22.5
1979 (est.)	7.8	1968	24.5
1978	9.6	1967	28.0
1977	11.2	1966	29.1
1976	12.3	1965	31.6
1975	12.8	1964	33.3
1974	14.6	1963	35.8
1973	15.2	1962	35.2
1972	18.8	1961	36.9
1971	18.8	1960	37.1
1970	21.5	1950	83.3

*From National Center for Health Statistics: Advance report of final natality statistics. 1981. *Monthly vital statistics report*. Vol. 29. No. 13 Public Health Service, Hyattsville, Md. Sept. 17, 1981.

8. Table 1-3, shows the selected infant mortality rates by age from 1950–1980.

   a. The infant mortality rate for under 28 days was _____ in 1950 and _____ in 1980.*

   b. In the 18 days to 11 months range there has been a consistently downward trend with the exception of which years? _____.*

   c. Briefly discuss inferential considerations of infant mortality rate.

9. Table 1-4, shows the maternal mortality from 1950–1980. For the most part, the rate becomes progressively lower.

   a. Identify the year(s) in which there was a deviation from this consistently downward trend. _____.*

   b. Briefly discuss inferential considerations of maternal mortality rate.

*These questions are addressed at the end of Part I.

Table 1–5. Birth Rates by Age of Mother, Live-Birth Order, and Race of Child, United States, 1980*

Live-birth order and race of child	Age of mother										
	15–44 years[1]	10–14 years	15–19 years			20-24 years	25-29 years	30-34 years	35-39 years	40-44 years	45-49 years
			Total	15-17 years	18-19 years						
All races											
Total	68.4	1.1	53.0	32.5	82.1	115.1	112.9	61.9	19.8	3.9	0.2
First child	29.5	1.1	41.4	28.5	59.7	57.3	38.2	12.8	2.6	0.3	0.0
Second child	21.8	0.0	9.8	3.6	18.6	39.8	41.9	20.7	4.2	0.5	0.0
White											
Total	64.7	0.6	44.7	25.2	72.1	109.5	112.4	60.4	18.5	3.4	0.2
First child	28.4	0.6	36.0	22.7	54.8	57.2	39.6	12.8	2.5	0.3	0.0
Second child	21.0	0.0	7.6	2.3	15.1	37.8	42.6	20.7	4.0	0.4	0.0
All other											
Total	88.6	3.9	94.6	68.3	133.2	145.0	115.5	70.8	27.9	6.5	0.4
First child	35.6	3.7	68.3	57.1	84.9	57.5	30.0	12.6	3.2	0.5	0.0
Second child	26.2	0.1	20.8	9.9	36.8	50.3	37.8	20.8	5.6	0.7	0.0
Black											
Total	88.1	4.3	100.0	73.6	138.8	146.3	109.1	62.9	24.5	5.8	0.3
First child	35.2	4.2	71.8	61.3	87.3	55.9	24.3	9.1	2.4	0.3	0.0
Second child	25.7	0.1	22.3	10.9	39.0	51.2	35.6	16.8	4.2	0.5	0.0

*Based on 100% of births in selected states and on a 50% sample of births in all other states. Rates are live births per 1000 women in specified age and racial groups. Live-birth order refers to number of children born alive to mother. Modified from National Center for Health Statistics: Advance report of final natality statistics. 1980. *Monthly vital statistics report*. Vol. 31, No. 8, Supp. DHHS Pub. No. (PHS) 83–1120. Public Health Service, Hyattsville, Md. November, 1982.
[1]Rates computed by relating total births, regardless of age of mother, to women aged 15–44 years.

10. Table 1-5 contains data about the ages at which mothers bear their first child.
   a. Identify the age at which the greatest number of women (of all races) have their first baby.

   _____.*

   b. Is this age the same for *white, black* and *all other* mothers? _____.*

11. What implications does the information in Tables 1-1, 1-2, and 1-3 have for identifying high-risk infants?

12. What implications does the information in Tables 1-4 and 1-5 have for identifying target groups for women's health care?

Family Dynamics

13. Define *family*.

*These questions are addressed at the end of Part I.

14. Discuss the factors that affect family structures.

    a.

    b.

    c.

15. Describe each of the following types of family configuration:

    a. Single adult living alone

    b. Nuclear dyad

    c. Single-parent family

    d. Nuclear family

    e. Three-generation family

f. Extended family (kin network)

g. Communal family

h. Homosexual family

i. Common-law family

16. Identify three functions of a family.
    a.

    b.

    c.

17. Define *role*.

18. Briefly describe the various roles a nurse assumes when working with families.

19. How may an individual's perception of an adult's role or a child's role influence the care that a childbearing family receives?

20. List and briefly explain eight of Duvall's family developmental tasks.

   a.

   b.

   c.

   d.

   e.

f.

g.

h.

21. Erikson has identified eight developmental stages. Each stage presents a core problem or conflict that must be resolved (at least to some degree) before an individual can progress to the subsequent stage. Complete the following chart of Erikson's stages:

STAGE	AVERAGE AGE	PRIMARY CONFLICT	ANTICIPATED BEHAVIORS

a.

b.

c.

d.

e.

f.

g.

h.

22. How might your knowledge of Duvall's and Erikson's theories influence your care of a childbearing family during the prenatal, intrapartal, postpartal, and neonatal periods?

Selected Answers

This section addresses the asterisked questions found in this chapter.

6. a. 8.5
   b. Other conditions originating in the perinatal period
   c. Certain gastrointestinal diseases; pneumonia and influenza
   d. They decreased.

7. b. Under 15 years of age; black (17.2).
   c. 25–29 years of age (5.8%).
   d. Yes; no (30–34 years of age).

8. a. 20.5 in 1950; 8.4 in 1980.
   b. 1975 and 1978.

9. a. 1963 (slight decrease, to 35.8); 1971–1972 (remained the same, at 18.8).

10. a. 18–19 years of age (59.7).
    b. No. The largest number of white women have their first child between the ages of 20 and 24. However, the largest number of black women and all other women have their first child between the ages of 18 and 19.

PART II
SELF-ASSESSMENT GUIDE

The following multiple-choice questions will help you assess your knowledge of the content of this chapter. Select the best answer for each of the questions and then refer to the end of Part II to check your answers.

1. Which of the following would be most qualified to provide ambulatory prenatal and postpartal care to a childbearing woman?

   a. Clinic nurse
   b. Obstetric nurse practitioner
   c. Lay midwife
   d. Acute-care clinical nurse specialist

2. Perinatal mortality is a combination of

   a. infant death rate and neonatal mortality.
   b. fetal death rate and infant death rate.
   c. neonatal mortality and postneonatal mortality.
   d. fetal death rate and neonatal mortality.

3. You are involved in a research project designed to determine whether patients seem to tolerate labor better if they are permitted to take a warm shower whenever they wish (provided their membranes are intact). In this case, you would be making use of the statistics you obtain to

    a. help establish a data base for different patient populations.
    b. provide information about your local maternity population.
    c. evaluate the success of specific nursing interventions.
    d. determine the level of patient care requirements.

4. Lisa and John and their 6-month-old son live in a duplex. Lisa's parents live in the other half of the duplex and are available any time for babysitting. In exchange, John maintains the yard and Lisa drives her mother to the doctor. What type of family configuration best describes this situation?

    a. Kin network
    b. Three-generation family
    c. Nuclear family
    d. Communal family

Carolyn and Earl Weaver were tired of listening to their children argue about curfew, church attendance, and assigned jobs, so they established a complaint box. Each family member may write up to one complaint per week. These are then drawn from the box and considered by all at a family meeting every Monday.

5. What family developmental task were the Weavers attempting to meet?

    a. Division of labor
    b. Placement of members into the larger society
    c. Socialization of family members
    d. Maintenance of order

6. Which family category best describes the Weavers?

    a. Traditional
    b. Democratic
    c. Authoritarian
    d. Liberated

7. Alexis, age 2½ years, is being potty trained. Her mother uses a great deal of positive reinforcement, and Alexis has made great progress. She hasn't had any wet pants during the day for the past six days and only occasionally wets at night. According to Erikson, what developmental stage is she in?

    a. Initiative vs. guilt
    b. Trust vs. mistrust
    c. Industry vs. inferiority
    d. Autonomy vs. shame and doubt

8. Which of the following best describes Erikson's developmental stage of identity vs. role confusion?

    a. Laura and Kevin have been dating for 9 months and recently became engaged.
    b. Martha is interested in teaching and spent the summer following her senior year of high school working as a camp counselor.
    c. Jon has worked as a systems analyst for 23 years. He recently returned to school for an advanced degree and now teaches parttime at the local community college.
    d. Following his retirement last year, Martin became active in the foster grandparent program in town and even encouraged two of his friends to join.

Answers

1.	b	5.	d
2.	d	6.	b
3.	c	7.	d
4.	a	8.	b

SELECTED BIBLIOGRAPHY

Aspy, V.H., and Roebuck, F.N. September-October 1979. Considering patient-centered obstetric nursing care: why and how? *J. Obstet. Gynecol. Neonatal Nurs.* 8:297.

Barnett, S.D., and Sellers, P. September-October 1979. Neonatal critical care nurse practitioner: a new role in neonatology. *MCN.* 4:279.

Beebe, J.E., and Thompson, H.O. May-June 1979. A paradigm of ethics for the maternal child nurse. *MCN.* 4:141.

Candy, M.M. March-April 1979. Birth of a comprehensive family-centered maternity program. *J. Obstet. Gynecol. Neonatal Nurs.* 8:80.

Davies, M., and Yoshida, M. March 1981. A model for cultural assessment. *Can. Nurse.* 77:22.

Friedman, M.M. 1981. *Family nursing theory and assessment.* New York: Appleton-Century-Crofts.

Grosso, C., et al. May-June 1981. The Vietnamese-American family . . . and grandma makes three. *MCN.* 6:177.

Hawkins, M.M. July-August 1980. Nursing and regionalization of perinatal services. *J. Obstet. Gynecol. Neonatal Nurs.* 9:215

Henderson, G., and Primeaux, M. 1981. *Transcultural health care.* Menlo Park, Calif.: Addison-Wesley Publishing Co.

Kuramoto, A.M., and Sandahl, B.B. March-April 1980. A quality assurance workshop for maternal child nurses. *MCN.* 5:87.

Layde, P.M., and Rubin, G.L. December 1982. Counting diseases and deaths meaningfully. *Contemp. OB/GYN.* 20:87.

Levine, N.H. March-April 1980. Family-centered maternity units: fact or fiction? *J. Obstet. Gynecol. Neonatal Nurs.* 9:116.

Maurice, S., and Warrick, L. November-December 1979. Ethics in professional nursing practice. *J. Obstet. Gynecol. Neonatal Nurs.* 8:327.

Meleis, A.I., and Sorrell, L. May-June 1981. Arab-American women and their birth experiences. *MCN.* 6:171.

Morrison, I., and Olsen, J. March 1979. Perinatal mortality and antepartum risk scoring. *Obstet. Gynecol.* 52:362.

Paukert, S.E. November-December 1979. One hospital's experience with implementing family-centered maternity care. *J. Obstet. Gynecol. Neonatal Nurs.* 8:351.

Shearer, M.H. Spring 1983. Not identifying the sources of the recent decline in perinatal mortality rates. *Birth.* 10:33.

Steinman, M.E., and Farr, J.D. July-August 1980. Nurse practitioner acceptance in private OB/GYN practice. *J. Obstet. Gynecol. Neonatal Nurs.* 9:240.

Stubblefield, P.G., and Berek, J.S. December 1980. Perinatal mortality in term and post-term births. *Obstet. Gynecol.* 56:676.

Whall, A.L. Oct. 1980. Congruence between existing theories of family functioning and nursing theories. *ANS* 3:59.

CHAPTER 2 # THE HUMAN REPRODUCTIVE SYSTEM

INTRODUCTION

The sexual development of males and females is both similar and different. During the first weeks following conception, it is impossible to determine the sex of the developing embryo. As gestation progresses, distinctions become more apparent. In most cases, the sexual characteristics develop normally, so that at birth the sex of the neonate is readily apparent. During the years that follow, the child learns the roles assigned to a male or female of the culture.

Puberty represents a major developmental milestone. Secondary sex characteristics develop, the reproductive organs mature, and the adolescent becomes capable of procreation.

This chapter focuses primarily on the reproductive system of both males and females. Subsequent chapters build on this knowledge and relate it to the entire process of procreation.

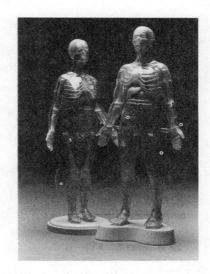

PART I
GENERAL PRINCIPLES AND CONCEPTS

Male Reproductive System

1. The male copulatory organ is the _____.

2. The shaft of the penis is composed of three columns of erectile tissue. The two lateral columns are

    called the _____; the third column, called the

    _____, contains the _____.

3. The distal end of the penis, analogous to the female clitoris, is termed the

    _____. It is covered by the _____, or

    foreskin, and may be removed surgically by circumcision.

4. Describe the appearance of the scrotum.

5. What is the primary function of the scrotum?

6. The scrotum is divided by a septum into two lateral compartments. Identify three structures of the male internal reproductive system that are found in each compartment.

    a.

    b.

    c.

7. What are two main functions of the testes?

    a.

    b.

8. The primary function of the epididymis is _____.

9. The primary function of the vas deferens (seminal duct) is _____.

10. The primary function of the seminal vesicles is _____.

11. The vas deferens and the duct of a seminal vesicle unite to form a short tube called the _____, which passes through the prostate gland and terminates in the urethra.

12. Briefly describe the location and primary function of the prostate gland.

13. What is the function of the alkaline secretion of the bulbourethral or Cowper's glands?

14. Label the parts of the male reproductive system indicated on Figure 2-1.

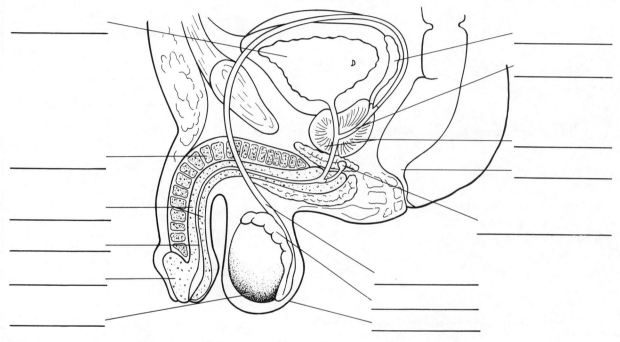

Figure 2-1. Male reproductive system.

15. Briefly describe the composition of semen.

16. The average volume of semen ejaculated after several days of sexual abstinence is
   _____ mL.

17. The normal sperm count per ejaculation is _____.

18. Sterility results with sperm counts less than _____.

Female Reproductive System

19. Identify the four bones of the human pelvis.

   a.

   b.

   c.

   d.

20. Identify the three main parts of each innominate bone.

   a.

   b.

   c.

21. Label the following structures on Figure 2-2:

Sacral body	Sacroiliac ligament
Left ileum	Sacrospinous ligament
Symphysis pubis	Sacrotuberous ligament
Right sacroiliac joint	

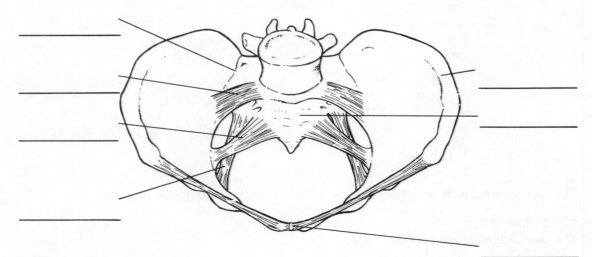

Figure 2-2.   Bony pelvis with ligaments.

22. Figure 2-3 focuses on the muscles of the pelvic floor. Label the following structures:

Vagina
Coccyx
Pubococcygeus muscle
Iliococcygeus muscle
Gluteus maximus muscle
Urogenital triangle (diaphragm)

Pudendal vessels
Bulbospongiosus muscle
External anal sphincter
Ischial tuberosity
Ischiocavernosus muscle
Adductor longus muscle

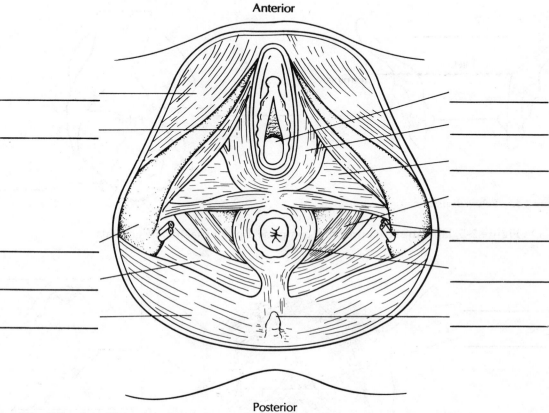

Figure 2-3. Muscles of the pelvic floor.

23. The major muscle group that forms the pelvic diaphragm is the _____.

24. Define the following terms:

a. False pelvis

b. True pelvis

c. Pelvic inlet

d. Pelvic outlet

25. On Figure 2-4, label the false pelvis, true pelvis, pelvic inlet, and pelvic outlet.

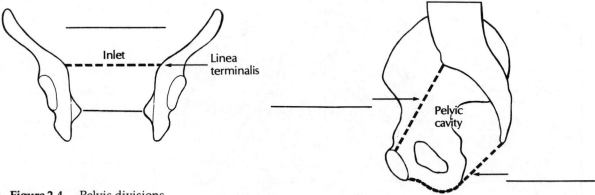

Figure 2-4. Pelvis divisions.

26. On Figure 2-5, label the structures that comprise the external female genitals.

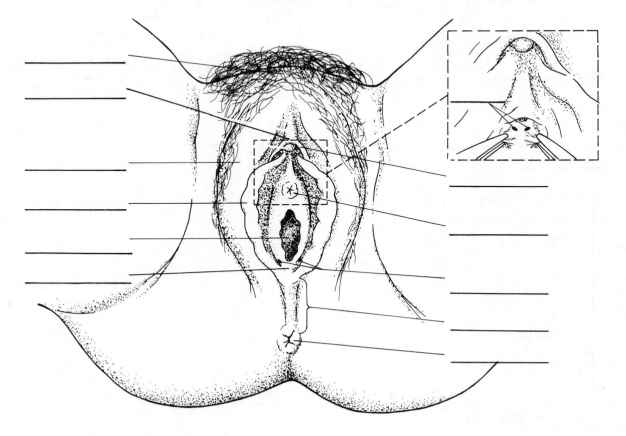

Figure 2-5. Female external genitals, longitudinal section.

27. State the function(s) of each of the following structures of the female external genitalia:

STRUCTURE   **FUNCTION**

Mons pubis

Labia majora

Labia minora

Clitoris

Urethral meatus

Paraurethral (Skene's)
  glands

Vaginal orifice (introitus)

Hymen

STRUCTURE   FUNCTION
Bartholin's glands

28. Figure 2-6 shows the female internal reproductive organs. Identify the structures that are indicated.

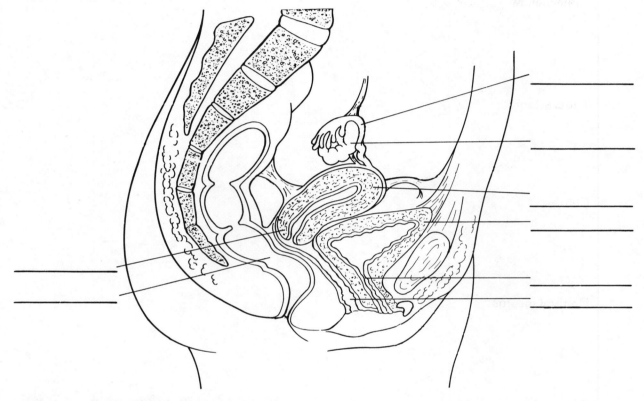

Figure 2-6.   Female internal reproductive organs.

29. Briefly discuss the function(s) of the vagina.

30. Name the four vaginal fornices and describe their location.

a.

b.

c.

d.

31. The pH of the vagina during a woman's reproductive years is _____.

32. Describe the shape and location of the uterus.

33. Label the uterine structures indicated in Figure 2-7.

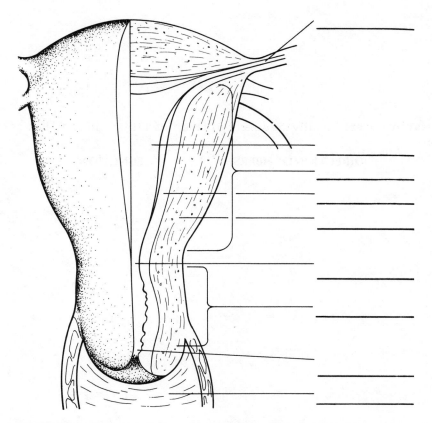

Figure 2-7. Anatomy of the uterus. (Modified from Spence, A.P., and Mason, E.B. 1983. *Human anatomy and physiology*, 2nd ed. Menlo Park, Calif.: Benjamin/Cummings Publishing Co., p. 742.)

34. How does the uterine cervix differ from the uterine corpus?

35. Identify three functions of the cervical mucosa.

    a.

    b.

    c.

36. The uterine musculature has three layers. Identify the direction of the muscle fibers in each layer and their primary function.

LAYER	DIRECTION OF FIBERS	FUNCTION
Outer		
Middle		
Inner		

37. The two main arteries supplying blood to the uterus and fallopian tubes are the
_____ and the _____.

38. Briefly describe the function of the endometrium.

39. Identify the location and function of each of the following uterine ligaments:

LIGAMENT	LOCATION	FUNCTION
Broad ligaments		
Round ligaments		
Cardinal ligaments		
Pubocervical ligaments		
Uterosacral ligaments		
Ovarian ligaments		

40. From what portion of the uterus do the fallopian tubes arise?

41. Identify the three parts of each fallopian tube.

    a.

    b.

    c.

42. What are the primary functions of the fallopian tubes?

43. In relation to the fallopian tubes, what is the purpose of each of the following?

    a. Fimbriae

b. Peristaltic movements

c. Nonciliated goblet cells of the mucosa

d. Tubal cilia

44. Briefly describe the appearance of the ovaries.

45. What is the primary function of the ovaries?

46. Define *Mittelschmerz*.

47. Label the major structures of the breast on Figure 2-8.

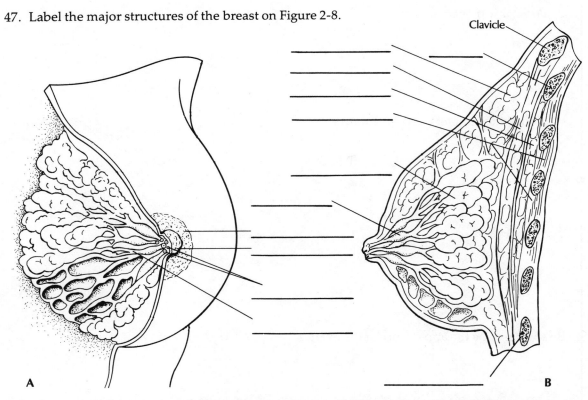

Clavicle

A

B

Figure 2-8. Anatomy of the breast. **A**, Anterior view of partially dissected left breast. **B**, Sagittal section. (Modified from Spence, A.P., and Mason, E.B. 1983. *Human anatomy and physiology*, 2nd ed. Menlo Park, Calif.: Benjamin/Cummings Publishing Co, p. 747.)

48. The nipple is composed primarily of _____ tissue.

49. What is the primary function of the tubercles of Montgomery?

Human Sexuality

50. Define the following terms and include a brief description of when or how each develops:

   a. Biologic sex

b. Sexual identity (core-gender identity)

c. Gender identity

d. Gender role behavior

51. Define *puberty*.

52. Briefly discuss the major physical changes that occur during puberty.

    a. Boys

    b. Girls

53. For each of the following hormones, state the source of secretion and the primary function(s).

HORMONE	SOURCE	FUNCTION
Testosterone		

HORMONE	SOURCE	FUNCTION
Estrogen		
Progesterone		
Follicle-stimulating hormone (FSH)		
Luteinizing hormone (LH)		
Prostaglandins (PGE and PGF$_{2\alpha}$)		

54. Define *menstruation*.

55. List the phases of the menstrual cycle and the days of occurrence of each.

   PHASE   **DAYS OF MENSTRUAL CYCLE**

56. Briefly describe the changes that occur in each of the following during the various phases of the menstrual cycle.

   a. Endometrium

   b. Cervical mucosa

   c. Ovarian follicle

57. Describe the process of ovulation.

58. Define *premenstrual tension*.

59. List the symptoms that may be associated with premenstrual tension.

60. How may premenstrual tension be managed?

61. Define the following terms:
    a. Amenorrhea

    b. Hypomenorrhea

    c. Hypermenorrhea

    d. Menorrhagia

    e. Metrorrhagia

    f. Dysmenorrhea

62. Define *coitus*.

63. Identify the four phases of sexual response described by Masters and Johnson.

    a.

    b.

    c.

    d.

64. Briefly describe the female and male sexual responses.

    a. Female

b. Male

Selected Answers

The questions in this chapter are factual, and the answers are readily available. Consequently, no questions were asterisked.

PART II
SELF-ASSESSMENT GUIDE

The following multiple-choice questions will help you assess your knowledge of the content of this chapter. Select the best answer for each of the questions and then refer to the end of Part II to check your answers.

1. The structure that provides a pathway for sperm to leave the epididymides is the

   a. vas deferens.
   b. dartos muscle.
   c. seminal vesicles.
   d. urethra.

2. The primary site of erotic sensation in the female reproductive tract is the

   a. mons pubis.
   b. vaginal introitus.
   c. labia minora.
   d. clitoris.

3. The normal position of the uterus is

   a. retroflexed.
   b. anteverted.
   c. vertical.
   d. none of the above.

4. The figure-eight pattern of the middle layer of uterine muscle fibers

   a. maintains the effects of uterine contractions during labor.
   b. differentiates the uterus into upper and lower segments.
   c. constricts large uterine vessels when the fibers contract.
   d. maintains uterine shape during pregnancy.

5. The ligaments that suspend the uterus from the lateral aspects of the true pelvis and provide the primary support for the uterus are the

   a. broad ligaments.
   b. cardinal ligaments.
   c. round ligaments.
   d. uterosacral ligaments.

6. What portion of the breast contains the cuboidal epithelial cells that secrete the components of milk?

   a. Alveoli
   b. Ducts
   c. Lactiferous sinuses
   d. Lobules

7. Which of the following situations best typifies gender identity?

   a. David, age 5½, refuses to wear a shirt he received that has pink dots on it. When asked why by his mother, he loudly proclaims: "Pink is for girls!"
   b. Mary, age 14, was born with normal external genitalia. Now she is in puberty, has secondary sex characteristics, and has fairly regular periods.
   c. Christie, age 25, has had several heterosexual relationships. She finds she is able to respond to sexual stimulation and achieves orgasm most of the time.
   d. Lyle, age 20, works with a highway construction crew during the summers. He is proud of his strength and endurance. During the school year, he attends college full time and is majoring in electrical engineering.

8. The structure that develops after rupture of the graafian follicle is the

   a. secondary follicle.
   b. zona pellucida.
   c. corpus luteum.
   d. corpus albicans.

9. Anne has very painful periods with excessively heavy menstrual flow. The terms that best describe her condition are

   a. dysmenorrhea and metrorrhagia.
   b. metrorrhagia and hypermenorrhea.
   c. amenorrhea and menorrhagia.
   d. dysmenorrhea and menorrhagia.

Answers

1. a   6. a
2. d   7. d
3. b   8. c
4. c   9. d
5. b

SELECTED BIBLIOGRAPHY

Beach, R.K. April 1982. Adolescent sexual decision making and sexual responsibility: perspectives for professionals in the 1980's. Paper presented at Adolescent Pregnancy: New Directions for the 80's, Rocky Mountain Chapter Society for Adolescent Medicine, Denver, Colorado.

Caldwell, B.V., and Behrman, H.R. 1981. Prostaglandins in reproductive processes. *Med. Clin. North Am.* 65(4):927.

Chihal, H.J. 1982. Painful periods and preludes. *Emergency Medicine* 14(17):33.

Dennerstein, L., et al. September 1980. Hormones and sexuality: effects of estrogen and progesterone. *Obstet. Gynecol.* 56:316.

Johnston, M. January-February 1980. Cultural variations in professional and parenting patterns. *J. Obstet. Gynecol. Neonatal Nurs.* 9:9.

Kuczynski, H.J. November-December 1980. Nursing and medical students' sexual attitudes and knowledge: curricular implications. *J. Obstet. Gynecol. Neonatal Nurs.* 9:339.

Leach, A.M. 1982. Threat to nurses' sexual identity. In *Comprehensive psychiatric nursing,* 2nd ed., ed. J. Haver, et al. New York: McGraw-Hill Book Co.

Leppink, M.A. Fall 1979. Adolescent sexuality. *Maternal-Child Nurs. J.* 8:153.

Page, E.W., et al. 1981. *Human reproduction: essentials of reproduction and perinatal medicine,* 3rd ed. Philadelphia: W.B. Saunders Co.

Pauerstein, C.S., and Eddy, C.A. April 1983. How the tubes function. *Contemp. OB/GYN.* 21:121.

Robertson, R.D., et al. December 1979. Assessment of ovulation by ultrasound and plasma estradiol determinations. *Obstet. Gynecol.* 54:686.

Urban, D.J., et al. May/June 1982. Nurse specialization in reproductive endocrinology. *J. Obstet. Gynecol. Neonatal Nurs.* 11(3):167.

Vijayakumar, R., et al. 1981. Myometrial prostaglandins during human menstrual cycle. *Am. J. Obstet. Gynecol.* 141(3):313.

Whitney, M.P., and Willingham, D. 1978. Adding a sexual assessment to the health interview. *J. Psychiatr. Nurs. Ment. Health Serv.* 16(4):17.

Zacharin, R.F. February 1980. Pulsion enterocele: review of functional anatomy of the pelvic floor. *Obstet. Gynecol.* 55:135.

CHAPTER 3 # CONCEPTION AND DEVELOPMENT OF THE HUMAN FETUS

INTRODUCTION

Conception and the development of a new being is a never-ending source of awe and fascination. As our knowledge of this process evolves, we develop greater insight into the potential ramifications of the physiologic, psychologic, and environmental factors that may impinge on it.

This chapter begins with a review of the process of conception. It then considers implantation, placental functioning, and fetal development. Factors that may influence fetal development are explored, with special emphasis on the impact of maternal medications.

This chapter's strong emphasis on anatomy and physiology provides a basis for subsequent chapters on the application of the nursing process for a childbearing family.

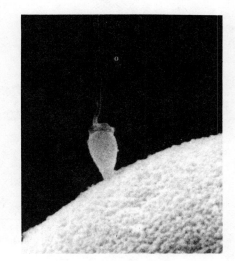

PART I
GENERAL PRINCIPLES AND CONCEPTS

1. Define the following terms:

   a. Gametes

   b. Chromosomes

   c. Autosomes

   d. Sex chromosomes

   e. Genes

    f. Homozygous genes

    g. Heterozygous genes

2. Compare mitosis and meiosis.

3. The normal sperm has _____ chromosomes.

4. The normal ovum has _____ chromosomes.

5. The normal infant has _____ chromosomes.

6. Which parent carries the chromosome that determines the sex of the child?

7. Define *ovum*.

8. What is the function of the flagellum of the sperm?

9. What portion of the sperm penetrates the ovum at the time of conception?

10. The sperm is viable for _____ hours after ejaculation.

11. The ovum is viable for _____ hours after ovulation.

12. Define *fertilization*.

13. The optimal place for fertilization to occur is _____.

14. What mechanism(s) is(are) involved in transporting the zygote (fertilized ovum) from the fallopian tube to the uterus?

15. Implantation occurs about _____ to _____ days after fertilization.

16. The zygote continually develops as it travels through the fallopian tube to its site of implantation in the uterus. Define the following terms, which relate to this developmental process:

   a. Zona pellucida

   b. Cleavage

   c. Blastomeres

   d. Morula

   e. Blastocysts

   f. Trophoblasts

17. Briefly describe how implantation occurs.

18. Define the following terms:

    a. Decidua

    b. Decidua capsularis

    c. Decidua basalis

    d. Decidua vera

19. Define each of the following stages of human development in utero:

    a. Embryo

    b. Fetus

20. Identify the three germ layers of the developing fetus and at least four structures derived from each layer.

    GERM LAYER   **DEVELOPING STRUCTURES**

    a.

    b.

    c.

21. Briefly describe the process by which the placenta develops.

22. Describe the general appearance of the placenta.

23. How does the maternal side of the placenta differ from the fetal side?

24. Identify three functions of the placenta.

   a.

   b.

   c.

25. List the four major placental hormones.

   a.

   b.

c.

d.

26. Prior to production of progesterone by the placenta, it is produced by the _____.

27. What is the purpose of the yolk sac during embryonic development?

28. The body stalk, which attaches the embryo to the yolk sac, develops into the _____.

29. The umbilical cord is made up of _____ vein(s), _____ artery (ies) and specialized connective tissue called _____.

Fetal Membranes

30. The embryonic membranes begin to form at the time of implantation. Two distinct membranes develop, the _____ and _____.

31. Describe the normal amount and composition of amniotic fluid.

32. List three functions of amniotic fluid.

a.

b.

c.

Fetal Circulation

33. Describe the function of each of the following fetal structures:

   a. Umbilical vein

   b. Ductus venosus

   c. Inferior vena cava

   d. Foramen ovale

   e. Ductus arteriosus

   f. Umbilical arteries

34. Label the following structures on Figure 3-1 and, using arrows, trace the normal pathway of fetal circulation:

Umbilical vein
Ductus venosus
Inferior vena cava
Foramen ovale
Ductus arteriosus
Umbilical arteries

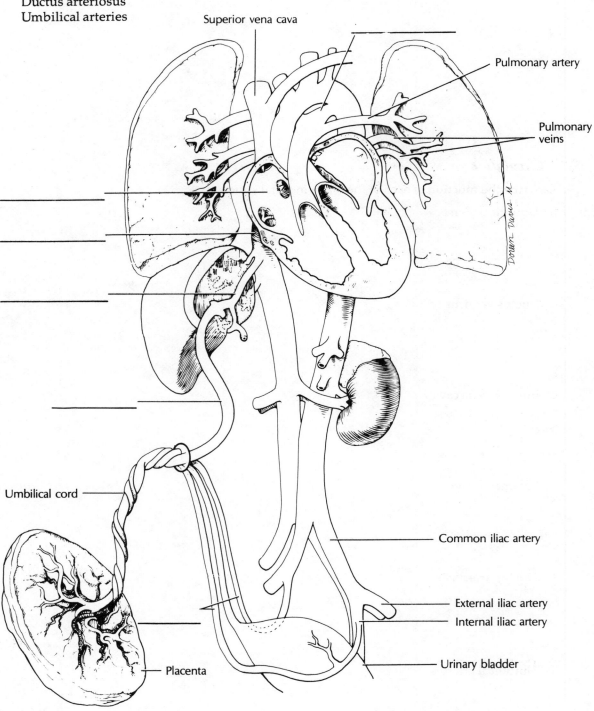

Superior vena cava

Pulmonary artery

Pulmonary veins

Umbilical cord

Common iliac artery

External iliac artery

Internal iliac artery

Urinary bladder

Placenta

Figure 3-1. Fetal circulation. (From Spence, A.P., and Mason, E.B. 1983. *Human anatomy and physiology,* 2nd ed. Menlo Park, Calif.: Benjamin/Cummings Publishing Co., p. 776.)

35. How does fetal circulation differ from infant and adult circulation?*

36. Complete the following chart of fetal development:

GESTATIONAL AGE	LENGTH	WEIGHT	ANATOMIC/PHYSIOLOGIC DEVELOPMENTAL CHANGES
4 weeks			
8 weeks			
12 weeks			
16 weeks			

*These questions are addressed at the end of Part I.

48

GESTATIONAL AGE	LENGTH	WEIGHT	ANATOMIC/PHYSIOLOGIC DEVELOPMENT CHANGES
20 weeks			
24 weeks			
28 weeks			
36 weeks			

37. Identify four factors that influence embryonic and fetal development.*

a.

b.

c.

d.

38. The fetus is most vulnerable to congenital malformation development during the first _____ weeks of life.

*These questions are addressed at the end of Part I.

39. Identify potential fetal problems that may develop for each of the following maternal medications:

MATERNAL MEDICATION	EFFECTS ON FETUS/NEONATE
Alcohol	
Estrogen	
Lysergic acid diethylamide (LSD)	
Phenobarbital	
Phenergan	
Progesterone	
Salicylate	
Tobacco	
Tetracycline	
Tolbutamide (Orinase)	

40. You are assisting in a prenatal class on fetal development. Mrs. Elizabeth Oliver, a 22-year-old primigravida, is 14 weeks pregnant and has the following questions. Based on your knowledge of fetal development, how would you respond?

   a. "When will my baby look like a baby?"

b. "How long is my baby now and how much does it weigh?"

c. "When will I feel my baby move?"

d. "When will my baby's heart start beating?"

e. "When can my baby's sex be identified?"

f. "Can my baby open its eyes?"

Selected Answers

This section addresses the asterisked questions found in this chapter.

35. Fetal circulation differs significantly from infant and adult circulation in that the fetus's oxygenated blood originates from the placenta and flows into the right atrium. It then moves through the foramen ovale (because of the low resistance on the left side of the fetal heart) and out the aorta to provide the head and upper body with highly oxygenated blood. Very little oxygenated blood flows into the lungs, because they are collapsed and offer a high resistance to blood flow. The blood that goes through the pulmonary artery is shunted into the aorta through the ductus arteriosus, bypassing the lungs to supply the rest of the body.

37. Many factors can influence the development of the embryo/fetus. Significant ones include the quality of the sperm or ova, teratogenic agents such as drugs and radiation, and maternal nutrition. Others you might have identified are any of the complications of pregnancy, such as maternal diabetes, hypertension, or TORCH infections.

PART II
SELF-ASSESSMENT GUIDE

The following multiple-choice questions will help you assess your knowledge of the content of this chapter. Select the best answer for each of the questions and then refer to the end of Part II to check your answers.

1. The mesoderm germ layer gives rise to the following structures:
   a. Alimentary canal, lungs, liver, and bladder
   b. Circulatory system, skin epithelium, and reproductive organs
   c. Muscles, lungs, and circulatory system
   d. Nervous system, lungs, and genitourinary system

2. The fetal sex organs have differentiated and are developed by the end of the

   a. first lunar month
   b. second lunar month.
   c. third lunar month.
   d. fourth lunar month.

3. The hormone that is primarily responsible for the maintenance of a pregnancy is

   a. estrogen.
   b. luteinizing hormone.
   c. progesterone.
   d. testosterone.

4. The morula, or "mulberry mass," is

   a. a small ball of cells.
   b. the differentiation of primary germ layers.
   c. the outer layer of cells replacing the zona pellucida.
   d. layers of cells surrounding a fluid-filled sac.

5. The chorion is

   a. a thin protective membrane containing amniotic fluid.
   b. the endometrium after implantation.
   c. the second cavity in the blastocyst.
   d. a thick membrane that develops from trophoblasts.

6. Nidation of the fertilized ovum occurs approximately how many days after conception?

   a. 3
   b. 5
   c. 7
   d. 9

7. The mature ovum is fertilizable for how many hours past ovulation?

   a. 8
   b. 12
   c. 24
   d. 36

8. At term, the placenta is

   a. composed of 15-20 cotyledons and weighs approximately 1/6 of the weight of the newborn.
   b. 6-8 inches in diameter and 1 inch thick and composed of 5-10 cotyledons.
   c. 2-4 inches in diameter and 1 inch thick at the center and weighs 1/5 of the weight of the newborn.
   d. composed of 10-15 cotyledons and 6-8 inches in diameter and ½ inch thick in the center.

9. A fetus weighing about 300 gm and measuring 18 cm in length that can actively suck and swallow amniotic fluid is approximately how many weeks gestation?

   a. 14 weeks
   b. 18 weeks
   c. 20 weeks
   d. 24 weeks

10. The functions of amniotic fluid include all of the following *except*

    a. controlling the embryonic/fetal temperature.
    b. protecting the fetus from injury.
    c. serving as a reservoir for fetal urine, epithelial cells, and albumin.
    d. nourishing the embryo/fetus.

Answers

1. c	6. c
2. c	7. c
3. c	8. a
4. a	9. c
5. d	10. d

SELECTED BIBLIOGRAPHY

Aladjen, S., and Lueck, J. 1982. Placental physiology. In *Gynecology and obstetrics,* ed. Sciarri, J.J. et al. Hogerstown, Md.: Harper & Row, Publishers, Inc.

Anderson, A.W., et al. September 1980. Biophysics of the developing heart, part I: the force-interval relationship. *Am. J. Obstet. Gynecol.* 138:33

Caffeine, cigarette smoke: effects on the unborn child. October 1980. *Hosp. Pract.* 15:160.

Charles, D. 1979. Placental transmission of antibiotics. *Obstet. Gynecol. Annu.* 8:19

Crelin, E.S. 1981. Development of the musculoskeletal system. *Clin. Symp. #1.* 33:2

Dilts, P.V. June 1981. Placental transfer. *Clin. Obstet. Gyne.* 24:555.

Elias, S., et al. September 1980. Genetic amniocentesis in twin gestations. *Am. J. Obstet. Gynecol.* 138:169.

Gusdon, J.P., and Sain, L.E. March 1981. Uterine and peripheral blood concentrations and human chorionic gonadotropin and human placental lactogen. *Am. J. Obstet. Gynecol.* 39:705.

Koffler, H. June 1981. Fetal and neonatal physiology. *Clin. Obstet. Gynecol.* 24:545.

McKay, S.R. January-February 1980. Smoking during the childbearing year. *MCN.* 5:46.

Naeye, R.L. December 1981. Maternal blood pressure and fetal growth. *Am. J. Obstet. Gynecol.* 141:780.

Nicholls, V., et al. June 1980. The influence of maternal factors on placental weight. *N.Z. Med. J.* 91:426.

Robinson, H.P., et al. December 1980. Diagnostic ultrasound: early detection of fetal neural tube defects. *Obstet. Gynecol.* 56:705.

Seeds, A.E. November 1980. Current concepts of amniotic fluid dynamics. *Am. J. Obstet. Gynecol.* 138:575.

Teasdale, F. July 1980. Gestational changes in the functional structure of the human placenta in relation to fetal growth: a morphometric study. *Am. J. Obstet. Gynecol.* 137:560.

Vorherr, H. March 1982. Factors influencing fetal growth. *Am. J. Obstet. Gynecol.* 142:577.

CHAPTER 4 ADAPTATIONS TO PREGNANCY

INTRODUCTION

During pregnancy, a woman's body undergoes a variety of changes designed to facilitate the growth and optimal maintenance of her developing fetus. Although the changes in her reproductive tract are the most dramatic, virtually all systems of her body are affected. In addition to physical changes, major psychologic changes occur as the couple adjusts to the fact that they will soon be parents.

This chapter focuses on the physical and psychologic changes that occur in preparation for childbirth. Subsequent chapters explore the nursing assessments and interventions that should accompany these changes.

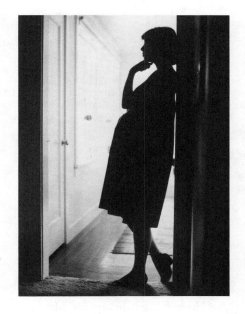

PART I
GENERAL PRINCIPLES AND CONCEPTS

Physical Adaptations to Pregnancy

1. Briefly describe changes in the size of the uterus that occur as a result of pregnancy.

2. Identify the major factors that contribute to the dramatic increase in uterine size.

3. How are the circulatory requirements of the uterus affected by pregnancy?

4. Describe the changes that occur in the cervical mucosa during pregnancy.

5. How is the mucous plug formed? What is its function?

6. How is ovum production affected by pregnancy?

7. What is the effect of pregnancy on the corpus luteum?

8. Briefly describe the vascular changes that occur in the vagina during pregnancy.

9. What is Chadwick's sign?

10. What is the significance of the increased acidity of the vaginal secretions during pregnancy?

11. Describe the breast changes that occur during pregnancy, with regard to the following:
    a. Size

   b. Pigmentation

   c. Montgomery's tubercles

   d. Formation and appearance of striae gravidarum

   e. Sensation

12. What is colostrum?

13. When does colostrum generally appear?

14. Why is there an increased tendency toward nasal stuffiness and epistaxis during pregnancy?

57

15. Briefly describe the changes that occur in the respiratory system during pregnancy.

16. How are the following components of the cardiovascular system affected by pregnancy?
    a. Blood volume

    b. Pulse rate

    c. Hemoglobin concentration

17. Explain the pseudoanemia frequently seen in pregnancy.

18. How is the bladder affected by the growing uterus?

19. What is the significance of the increase in the glomerular filtration rate that occurs during pregnancy?

20. How is gastric acidity affected by pregnancy?

21. What is the cause of "heartburn" during pregnancy?

22. Why does bloating and constipation occur during pregnancy?

23. Why do hemorrhoids more commonly occur during pregnancy?

24. Define and explain the following changes that may occur in the skin:

    a. Striae gravidarum

    b. Chloasma

    c. Linea nigra

    d. Spider nevi

25. Describe the functions of the following placental hormones:

    a. Human chorionic gonadotropin (hCG)

    b. Estrogen

    c. Progesterone

   d. Human placental lactogen (hPL)

26. Describe the effects of pregnancy on the following components of the endocrine system:

   a. Thyroid

   b. Parathyroid

   c. Pituitary

   d. Adrenals

27. What is the average weight gain during each trimester of pregnancy?

   a. First trimester: _____

   b. Second trimester: _____

   c. Third trimester: _____

28. Why does water retention commonly occur during pregnancy?

29. How is the metabolism of the following substances affected by pregnancy?

   a. Protein

   b. Carbohydrates

   c. Fats

   d. Minerals

30. Indicate when the following signs of pregnancy occur and identify them as presumptive, probable, or positive. For those signs that are presumptive or probable, indicate other causative factors.

	TIME OF APPEARANCE	PRE-SUMP-TIVE	PROB-ABLE	POSI-TIVE	OTHER CAUSATIVE FACTORS
Enlarging abdomen					
Goodell's sign					
Braxton Hicks con-tractions					
Fetal heart sounds					
Excessive fatigue					

	TIME OF APPEARANCE	PRE-SUMP-TIVE	PROB-ABLE	POSI-TIVE	OTHER CAUSATIVE FACTORS
Positive pregnancy test					
Fetal skeleton visible on x-ray film					
Nausea and vomiting					
Urinary frequency					
Breast changes					
Fetal movements					
Chadwick's sign					
Skin pigmentation changes					
Hegar's sign					
Amenorrhea					
Quickening					
Ladin's sign					

31. How would you explain the differences among presumptive, probable, and positive signs of pregnancy to an expectant mother?

32. Briefly describe each of the following pregnancy tests:

    IMMUNOASSAY

    a. Hemagglutination-inhibition test (Pregnosticon R)

    b. Latex agglutination tests (Gravidex and Pregnosticon slide test)

    c. Solid-phase radioimmune assay (hCG and Preg/Statβ-hCG)

    RADIORECEPTOR ASSAY

    a. Radioreceptor assay (Biocept G)

33. What factors may influence the reliability of a pregnancy test?

34. Why is a positive pregnancy test *not* a positive sign of pregnancy?

35. What factors contribute to false readings in using over-the-counter pregnancy tests?*

Psychologic Adaptation to Pregnancy

36. The reaction of many women to a confirmation of pregnancy is "someday but not now." Why are feelings of ambivalence a common reaction to pregnancy?

37. Briefly summarize behaviors that are commonly seen in each trimester as a woman adjusts to pregnancy.

TRIMESTER	BEHAVIORS
First trimester	

*These questions are addressed at the end of Part I.

TRIMESTER	BEHAVIORS
Second trimester	
Third trimester	

38. Discuss the possible effects of pregnancy on a woman's body image.*

39. Discuss the reactions of expectant fathers to pregnancy with regard to the following:
   a. Role change

   b. Feelings of rivalry with and resentment toward his pregnant partner.

*These questions are addressed at the end of Part I.

c. *Mitleiden*

d. Rehearsing for fatherhood

Selected Answers

This section addresses the asterisked questions found in this chapter.

35. False results may occur with over-the-counter pregnancy tests if a test is performed too soon after a missed period. (Some tests require waiting until the ninth day; others may be done by the sixth day after a missed period.)

    False readings may also occur if a specimen other than the first of the day is used, because the first specimen contains the highest levels of hCG.

    Other factors that may contribute to a false reading include a dirty kit or a kit containing traces of soap or detergent, exposure of the sample to heat or sunlight, a sample that has stood longer than the specified time period, or movement of the test-tube sample during the timing period.

38. The effects of pregnancy on a woman's body image are greatly influenced by her feelings about her pregnancy and by cultural, physiologic, psychosocial, and interpersonal factors. Although the classic idea of the "glow of pregnancy"—a woman at her most lovely—has romantic appeal, it isn't necessarily true. When it does occur, it is most frequently seen in the second trimester when a woman has begun wearing maternity clothes. In the last weeks of pregnancy, a woman may feel constantly tired and misshapen and may, as a result, have a negative body image.

    You are on the right track if you recognized that a variety of factors influence body image and that, although there is no one correct answer, certain types of responses occur frequently.

PART II
SELF-ASSESSMENT GUIDE

The following multiple-choice questions will help you assess your knowledge of the content of this chapter. Select the best answer for each of the questions and then refer to the end of Part II to check your answers.

1. The primary cause of uterine enlargement during pregnancy is the

    a. engorgement of preexisting vascular structures.
    b. formation of an additional layer of uterine musculature.
    c. hypertrophy of preexisting myometrial cells.
    d. increased number of myometrial cells.

2. During the first 10-12 weeks of pregnancy, the corpus luteum

   a. gradually regresses and becomes obliterated.
   b. secretes estrogen to maintain the pregnancy.
   c. secretes human chorionic gonadotropin to maintain the pregnancy.
   d. secrets progesterone to maintain the pregnancy.

3. During pregnancy, the increased number and activity of the endocervical glands are responsible for

   a. a marked softening of the cervix.
   b. a thiner, more watery mucosal discharge.
   c. the development of Chadwick's sign.
   d. the formation of the mucous plug.

4. The pseudoanemia of pregnancy is related to a decreased hematrocrit, which is caused by

   a. a greater increase in plasma volume than in hemoglobin levels.
   b. decreased hemoglobin levels.
   c. a decrease in both plasma volume and hemoglobin levels.
   d. increased plasma volume without any concurrent increase in hemoglobin levels.

5. Which of the following hormones is similar to the growth hormone in function and also contributes to the rise in blood glucose levels during pregnancy?

   a. Estrogen
   b. HCG
   c. HPL
   d. Progesterone

6. All of the following factors contribute to fluid retention during pregnancy *except*

   a. decreased tubular reabsorption in the kidneys.
   b. increased levels of adrenocorticosteroids.
   c. increased venous stasis in the lower extremities.
   d. lowered serum protein levels.

7. Constipation during pregnancy is usually the result of

   a. prolonged stomach emptying time and decreased intestinal motility.
   b. increased peristalsis and flatulence.
   c. increased cardiac workload resulting in delayed peristalsis.
   d. reflux of acidic gastric contents and hypochlorhydria.

8. Over-the-counter pregnancy tests determine the presence of hCG in the woman's

   a. blood.
   b. saliva.
   c. urine.
   d. vaginal secretions.

9. All of the following statements describe normal psychologic changes during pregnancy *except*

   a. a woman's emotions are labile and mood swings are common.
   b. changes in body image occur as a result of a variety of physical, psychosocial, and cultural factors.
   c. feelings of ambivalence about pregnancy indicate probable mothering problems following delivery.
   d. introversion or an inward focusing on oneself may cause an outgoing woman to appear more quiet and reserved.

Answers

1. c   6. a
2. d   7. a
3. d   8. c
4. a   9. c
5. c

SELECTED BIBLIOGRAPHY

Admire, G., and Byers, L. April 1981. Counseling the pregnant teenager. *Nurs. 81.* 11:62.

Bartel, C.H. March 1981. Old enough to get pregnant . . .too young to have babies. *Nurs. 81.* 11:44.

Briggs, E. Summer 1979. Transition to parenthood. *Maternal-Child Nurs. J.* 8:69.

Lumley, J. Spring 1980. The image of the fetus in the first trimester: what the mother thinks about the fetus. *Birth Fam. J.* 7:5.

Porter, L.S., and Demeuth, B.R. Summer 1979. The impact of marital adjustment on pregnancy acceptance. *Maternal-Child Nurs. J.* 8:103.

Quagliorello, J., et al. January 1979. Relaxin secretion in early pregnancy. *Obstet. Gynecol.* 53:62.

Rich, C. Fall 1979. A multigravida's work at organizing during pregnancy. *Maternal-Child Nurs. J.* 8:195.

Soules, M.R., et al. June 1980. Nausea and vomiting of pregnancy: role of human chorionic gonadotropin and 17-hydroxyprogesterone. *Obstet. Gynecol.* 55:696.

Zlatnik, F.V., et al. August 1979. Human placental lactogen: a predictor of perinatal outcome? *Obstet. Gynecol.* 54:205.

CHAPTER 5 *NURSING ASSESSMENT AND CARE OF THE ANTEPARTAL FAMILY*

INTRODUCTION

The antepartal period is a time of great significance for both the expectant family and the unborn child. During this time, the family must adjust to the physical and psychologic changes occurring in the mother and must also come to terms with the impact a new baby will have on their own lives and roles. Nurses caring for the antepartal family must primarily consider the mother and her unborn child but cannot neglect the father, siblings, and others who form a significant part of the mother's support system.

For the fetus, this is a time of unparalleled growth and development but also a time when his well-being is directly related to his mother's health, personal habits, and environment.

Accurate, concise assessment forms the basis for effective antepartal care. Once a complete assessment has been made, needs and problems can be identified, and the nurse can work with the patient to formulate a plan of care to meet these needs. Without patient input and compliance, even the best-formulated plan has little chance of succeeding. An ongoing process of evaluation then becomes necessary to modify the plan as the pregnancy progresses.

This chapter is designed to assist you in identifying common antepartal changes and health needs so that you may use this knowledge in assessing antepartal families and in planning, implementing, and evaluating their care.

PART I
GENERAL PRINCIPLES AND CONCEPTS

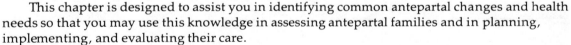

1. Define the following terms, which are used when developing a client's obstetric history:

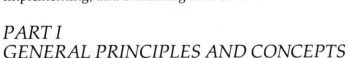

   a. Gravida

   b. Primigravida

    c. Multigravida

    d. Para

    e. Nullipara

    f. Primipara

    g. Multipara

    h. Abortion

    i. Stillbirth

    j. Gestation

2. Alexis Page is pregnant for the fourth time. She lost her first pregnancy at 12 weeks' gestation. She has two children at home. How would you record her obstetric history?

Gravida _____   Para _____   Ab _____

3. Martha Davies is pregnant for the third time. She delivered a stillborn fetus at 37 weeks' gestation and has a 3-year-old at home. How would you record her obstetric history?

Gravida _____   Para _____   Ab _____

4. The following questionnaire is similar to many that are used when a woman initially seeks antepartal care. With a friend or family member acting as the client and you as the prenatal nurse, obtain the necessary information. (Note: This questionnaire focuses primarily on factors related to pregnancy and is not a complete history of all body systems.)*

Name: _____ Age: _____ Race: _____

Address: _____ Phone: _____

Educational Level: _____ Occupation: _____

Marital Status: _____

Have any members of your family had the following? If so, who?

_____ Diabetes _____

_____ Cardiovascular disease _____

_____ High blood pressure _____

_____ Breast cancer _____

_____ Other types of cancer _____

_____ Multiple pregnancies _____

_____ Preeclampsia-eclampsia _____

_____ Congenital anomalies _____

*These questions are addressed at the end of Part I.

How old were you when your menstrual periods started? _____

How often do they occur? _____

How long do they last? _____

Do you have any discomfort with your periods? _____ If so, how severe is it? _____

What is the date of the first day of your last normal menstrual period? _____

Have you had any bleeding or spotting since your last normal menstrual period? _____

Have you had any of the following diseases?

_____ Chickenpox	_____ Asthma
_____ Mumps	_____ High blood pressure
_____ Three-day measles (rubella)	_____ Heart disease
_____ Two-week measles (rubeola)	_____ Respiratory disease
_____ Kidney disease	_____ Diabetes
_____ Frequent bladder infections	_____ Allergies
_____ Thyroid problems	_____ Venereal disease
_____ Anemia	_____ Other

(If client answers *yes* to any of the above, include pertinent information in this space.)

Have you been on birth control pills? _____ If yes, when did you stop taking them? _____

Were you using any other method of contraception? _____ If so, what method? _____

How many previous pregnancies have you had? _____

Have you had any miscarriages or abortions? _____ If yes, how many? _____

How many living children do you have? _____

Have you had any stillbirths? _____ If yes, how many? _____

Gravida _____   Para _____   Ab _____

Previous children:

Date of birth	*Sex*	*Birthweight*	*Premature or full term*
1.			
2.			
3.			
4.			
5.			

Did any previous children have problems immediately after birth? _____ If yes, what occurred?

Have you had any problems with previous pregnancies? _____ If yes, what occurred?

Have you had any problems with previous labors and/or deliveries? _____ If yes, what occurred?

Have you had any problems with previous postpartal periods? _____ If yes, what occurred?

Are you presently taking any prescription or nonprescription drugs? _____ If yes, please list them.

1.   3.

2.   4.

Do you smoke? _____ Number of cigarettes per day: _____

How much of the following do you drink per day?

1. Coffee _____

2. Tea _____

3. Colas _____

4. Alcoholic beverages _____

What is your present weight? _____

What is your usual pre-pregnant weight? _____

Nursing assessment of available psychosocial data (to be completed by nurse using information obtained from the patient or other sources):**

**This should be a brief summary of your impression of the client, her ability to cope with her pregnancy, plans she has made, and available support systems.

Brief description of available support persons (include marital status and information about the father of the child, such as age, occupation, involvement in the pregnancy):

Client feelings about the pregnancy.

Plans for adapting to the pregnancy:

5. The following blood tests are frequently done during the initial physical exam. List the normal findings and the rationale for doing each.

TEST	NORMAL FINDINGS	RATIONALE
Serology		
Hematocrit		
Hemoglobin		

TEST	NORMAL FINDINGS	RATIONALE
White blood cells (WBC)		
ABO and Rh typing		
Rubella titer		

6. A urinalysis and urine culture and sensitivity are also done. What types of abnormal findings are possible and what is their significance?

The procedure for a complete physical examination may be reviewed in textbooks on physical assessment. This workbook focuses on those aspects of the physical examination that are directly related to assessment of the pregnancy.

7. Allison Scott, gravida I para 0 ab 0, is scheduled for her first obstetric examination. Identify three areas of focus in this examination.*

   a.

   b.

   c.

*These questions are addressed at the end of Part I.

8. During her examination, the doctor measures Allison's fundal height. How is this measured?

9. What information does fundal height provide about the pregnancy?

10. Allison asks you when the baby's heartbeat will be heard. When is the fetal heartbeat usually detected?

   a. With a fetoscope: _____

   b. With a doppler: _____

11. To complete a pelvic examination, Allison is placed in the _____ position.

12. Identify the three basic parts of every initial pelvic examination.*

   a.

   b.

   c.

13. State Nägele's rule.

*These questions are addressed at the end of Part I.

14. Allison began her last normal menstrual period on May 28 of this year. Using Nägele's rule, calculate her expected date of confinement (EDC).

15. What is the recommended frequency of prenatal visits for a normal prenatal client?

16. Identify the factors that you would consider as part of your initial psychologic assessment of an antepartal family.

17. What behaviors might indicate psychologic problems in relation to the pregnancy?

18. The following chart lists discomforts that commonly occur during pregnancy. For each discomfort, briefly describe the cause and possible interventions for alleviating it.

DISCOMFORT	TIME OF OCCURRENCE	CAUSE	METHODS OF ALLEVIATION
Nausea/ vomiting			
Urinary frequency and urgency			
Breast tenderness			
Fatigue			
Increased vaginal discharge			
Heartburn			
Ankle edema			
Varicose veins			
Hemor- rhoids			
Constipa- tion			
Backache			
Leg cramps			
Faintness			
Shortness of breath			

19. Allison Scott is interested in breast-feeding her baby and asks if there is anything she should do during pregnancy to prepare her breasts. What advice would you give her?

20. What advice would you give a pregnant woman who asks about the types of physical activity she may engage in during pregnancy?*

21. What changes in sexual desire and response frequently occur during pregnancy?

22. Allison asks about sexual intercourse during the third trimester. What information would you give her?

*These questions are addressed at the end of Part I.

23. During Allison's initial prenatal visit, you discuss the danger signals of pregnancy with her. Identify at least eight danger signals and explain the possible significance of each.

    DANGER SIGNAL   **SIGNIFICANCE**

    a.

    b.

    c.

    d.

    e.

    f.

    g.

    h.

24. What will you instruct Allison to do if she should experience any of the danger signals?

25. In counseling pregnant clients about their activities, what information would you provide about the following?

    a. Appropriate prenatal exercises

b. Medications

c. Dental care

d. Alcohol

e. Smoking

f. Caffeine

g. Social drugs

Nutrition and Pregnancy

26. Diana Cooper, a 22-year-old primipara, 2 months pregnant, is discussing nutrition with you. She is of normal weight and is very concerned about avoiding excessive weight gain. What pattern of weight gain would you recommend for her?

27. To achieve this weight gain, how much should she increase her caloric intake? _____

28. What are the functions of the following categories of nutrients?

    a. Protein

    b. Fats

    c. Carbohydrates

29. For each of the following vitamins or minerals, briefly describe its functions and identify some common food sources:

VITAMIN/MINERAL	FUNCTION	SOURCES
Vitamin A		
Vitamin D		

VITAMIN/MINERAL	FUNCTION	SOURCES
Vitamin E		
Vitamin K		
Vitamin C		
Thiamine (B_1)		
Riboflavin (B_2)		
Niacin		
Folic acid		
Pantotheric acid		

VITAMIN/MINERAL	FUNCTION	SOURCES
Pyridoxin (B_6)		
Cobalamin (B_{12})		
Calcium		
Phosphorus		
Iodine		
Sodium		
Zinc		

VITAMIN/MINERAL	FUNCTION	SOURCES
Magnesium		
Iron		

30. Tina Nelson is a true vegetarian and will not eat any food from animal sources, including milk and eggs. What foods might she use to meet her protein and calcium requirements during pregnancy?*

Psychologic Aspects of Care

31. What psychosocial factors might influence a woman during pregnancy?

32. Briefly discuss the psychologic tasks a woman must undertake during pregnancy.*

*These questions are addressed at the end of Part I.

33. Your close friend Lois has just received confirmation that she is 10 weeks pregnant. While visiting, she tells you that she feels some ambivalence about being pregnant and having a child, even though the pregnancy was planned. How might you respond?*

34. Describe the common reactions of expectant fathers during the course of a pregnancy.

35. Monica Clark is 6 months pregnant and asks for advice about how to prepare her 3-year-old son, Jared, for the birth of a sibling. What suggestions might you give her?

Preparation for Childbirth

36. Give a brief description of each of the following methods of childbirth preparation:

    a. Read method

*These questions are addressed at the end of Part I.

b. Psychoprophylactic method (Lamaze)

c. Bradley method

d. Hypnosis

e. Other (method commonly used in your area, if applicable)

Selected Answers

This section addresses the asterisked questions found in this chapter.

4. Taking an obstetric health history should help you focus on the information that is pertinent to high-quality maternity care. You should be able to identify a reason for each of the questions asked. You should also be able to identify information that may place a client in the high-risk category. In addition to such obvious problems as preexisting medical conditions, think about maternal age, weight, occupation, and previous obstetric history; family history of disorders; marital status and support system; smoking and alcohol consumption; and so on. Once you begin to recognize risk factors, you will be better able to plan for appropriate antepartal care.

7. The initial obstetric examination focuses on
   a. inspection, auscultation, and palpation of the abdomen.
   b. determination of the adequacy of the pelvis.
   c. vaginal examination.

12. The initial pelvic examination should include
   a. a Pap smear and any other pertinent cultures or smears.
   b. visual inspection of the external genitalia, vagina, and cervix.
   c. a bimanual examination.

20. Opinion varies about the amount of exercise advisable during pregnancy. In an uncomplicated pregnancy, clients may continue sports activities at which they are adept, especially during the early months. Some physicians express concern about the possibility of falling in sports such as skiing, bike riding, or tennis when the woman's abdomen enlarges and her center of gravity changes. If sports activities are of special importance to a woman, it is advisable for her to select a physician who has views that are acceptable to her.

30. In addition to the *frequently* used soybean products (soybean milk, curd, and so on), nuts, and lentils, pregnant vegetarians might include such protein sources as tofu in their diets. Possible additional sources of calcium include turnip greens, white beans, and almonds.

32. The first developmental task of the pregnant woman is to accept the pregnancy. Once this is achieved, the woman must come to accept her unborn child as distinct from herself. She must also accept the termination of pregnancy with the resulting physical separation from the fetus. During pregnancy, the woman begins the bonding process and starts to accept the mother role. She must also resolve any fears she may have about childbirth in order to cope effectively. You have probably noted things in the conversation or behavior of pregnant clients or friends that suggested that they were dealing with these developmental tasks.

33. We hope you told your friend that, even in the most desired pregnancy, feelings of ambivalence are normal. Role changes, physical changes, altered relationships, added financial responsibilities, and attitudes about parenting and values all affect a woman's, indeed a couple's, response to pregnancy.

PART II
SELF ASSESSMENT GUIDE

The following multiple-choice questions will help you assess your knowledge of the content of this chapter. Select the best answer for each of the questions and then refer to the end of Part II to check your answers.

1. Molly Higgins is pregnant again. She has two living children at home. A third child died of birth defects at 4 days of age. She has never had an abortion. Which of the following most accurately describes her now?

   a. Gravida III para II ab 0
   b. Gravida III para III ab 0
   c. Gravida IV para II ab I
   d. Gravida IV para III ab 0

2. Molly has a hemoglobin of 12.9 gm/dL and a hematocrit of 41%. Which of the following statements about these values is most accurate?

   a. Both are within normal limits.
   b. Hemoglobin is normal; hematocrit indicates a physiologic anemia.
   c. Hemoglobin indicates an iron-deficiency anemia; hematocrit is normal.
   d. Hemoglobin and hematocrit are elevated and indicate polycythemia.

3. Molly began her last normal menstrual period on November 19, 1983. Her estimated date of confinement (EDC) is

   a. August 12, 1984.
   b. August 26, 1984.
   c. September 16, 1984.
   d. September 19, 1984.

4. All of the common discomforts of pregnancy listed below generally have their initial onset during the second half of pregnancy *except*

   a. backache.
   b. dyspnea.
   c. fatigue.
   d. varicose veins.

5. Your friend is in her early months of pregnancy and complains about morning sickness. Which of the following recommendations might you make to her?

   a. Nothing will alleviate it, and you must do your best to accept it.
   b. Eat a dry carbohydrate, such as crackers, before arising.
   c. Take large quantities of fluids with meals.
   d. Eat three meals per day and avoid eating between meals.

6. All of the following are helpful in preparing the nipples of a pregnant woman who plans to breast-feed her baby *except*

   a. rolling each nipple between thumb and forefinger for a few minutes daily.
   b. washing the breasts and nipples thoroughly with soap and water each day.
   c. rubbing the nipples with a soft towel after her daily bath.
   d. encouraging oral stimulation of her nipples by her sexual partner during foreplay.

7. Which of the following symptoms should a woman be instructed to report to her health care provider immediately?

   a. Ankle edema
   b. Heartburn
   c. Urinary frequency
   d. Vaginal bleeding

8. The major developmental task that the mother must accomplish during the first trimester of pregnancy is

   a. acceptance of the pregnancy.
   b. acceptance of the termination of the pregnancy.
   c. acceptance of the fetus as a separate and unique being.
   d. satisfactory resolution of fears related to giving birth.

9. Which of the following menus would provide the highest amounts of protein, iron, and vitamin C?

   a. 4 oz beef, ½ c lima beans, a glass of skim milk, and ¾ c strawberries
   b. 3 oz chicken, ½ c corn, a lettuce salad, and a small banana
   c. 1 c macaroni, ¾ c peas, a glass of whole milk, and a medium pear
   d. A scrambled egg, a hash-browned potato, half a glass of buttermilk, and a large nectarine

10. All of the following are components of the psychoprophylactic (Lamaze) method of childbirth preparation *except*

    a. conditioned responses.
    b. breathing techniques for labor.
    c. active relaxation.
    d. planned self-hypnosis.

Answers

1.	d	6.	b
2.	a	7.	d
3.	b	8.	a
4.	c	9.	a
5.	b	10.	d

SELECTED BIBLIOGRAPHY

Abrams, B. March 1981. Helping pregnant teenagers eat right. *Nurs. 81.* 11:46.

Ashley, M. 1981. Alcohol use during pregnancy: a challenge for the 80s. *Can. Med. Assoc. J.* 125(2):141.

Baranowski, E. March-April 1983. Childbirth education classes for expectant deaf parents. *MCN.* 8(2):143.

Becker, C.H. November-December 1982. Comprehensive assessment of the healthy gravida. *J. Obstet. Gynecol. Neonatal Nurs.* 11(6):375.

Blum, R.W., and Goldhagen, J. May 1981. Teenage pregnancy in perspective. *Clin. Pediatr.* 20:335.

Bonovich, L. March-April 1981. Participation: the key to learning for patients in antepartal clinics. *J. Obstet. Gynecol. Neonatal Nurs.* 10:75.

Cameron, J. November-December 1979. Year-long classes for couples becoming parents. *MCN.* 4:358.

Carter-Jessop, L. March-April 1981. Promoting maternal attachment through prenatal intervention. *MCN.* 6:107.

Ellis, D.J. September-October 1980. Sexual needs and concerns of expectant parents. *J. Obstet. Gynecol. Neonatal Nurs.* 9:306.

Genest, M. March-April 1981. Preparation for childbirth, evidence for efficacy: a review. *J. Obstet. Gynecol. Neonatal Nurs.* 10:82.

Harris, R., et al. July-August 1980. Therapeutic uses of human figure drawings by the pregnant couple. *J. Obstet. Gynecol Neonatal Nurs.* 9:232.

Hogan, L. May-June 1979. Pregnant again—at 41. *MCN.* 4:174.

Jimenez, S.L.M. March-April 1980. Education for the childbearing year: comprehensive application of psychoprophylaxis. *J. Obstet. Gynecol. Neonatal Nurs.* 9:97.

Jimenez, S.M., et al. September-October 1979. Prenatal classes for repeat parents: a distinct need. *MCN.* 4:305.

Johnson, J.M. March-April 1980. Teaching self-hypnosis in pregnancy, labor and delivery. *MCN.* 5:98.

Josten, L. March-April 1981. Prenatal assessment guide for illuminating possible problems with parenting. *MCN.* 6:113.

Lamb, G.S., and Lipkin, M., Jr. March-April 1982. Somatic symptoms of expectant fathers. *MCN.* 7:110.

Lemasters, G.K. March-April 1981. Zinc insufficiency during pregnancy: a review. *J. Obstet. Gynecol. Neonatal Nurs.* 10:124.

Olson, B.K. March-April 1981. Patient comfort during pelvic examination: new foot support vs. metal stirrups. *J. Obstet. Gynecol. Neonatal Nurs.* 10:104.

Rang, M.L. January-February 1980. Bibliography for nutrition in pregnancy. *J. Obstet. Gynecol. Neonatal Nurs.* 9:55.

Swanson, J. September-October 1980. The marital relationship during pregnancy. *J. Obstet. Gynecol. Neonatal Nurs.* 9:267.

Sweet, P.T. March-April 1979. Prenatal classes especially for children. *MCN.* 4:82.

Tilden, V.P. January-February 1983. Perceptions of single vs. partnered adult gravidas in the midtrimester. *J. Obstet. Gynecol. Neonatal Nurs.* 12(1):40.

Tipping, V.G. Spring 1981. The vulnerability of a primipara during the antepartal period. *Maternal-Child Nurs. J.* 10:61.

Whitley, N. March-April 1979. A comparison of prepared childbirth couples and conventional prenatal class couples. *J. Obstet. Gynecol. Neonatal Nurs.* 8:109.

Woolery, L., and Barkley, N. May-June 1981. Enhancing couple relationships during prenatal and postnatal classes. *MCN.* 6:184.

Worthington-Roberts, B., and Weigle, A. January-February 1983. Caffeine and pregnancy outcome. *J. Obstet. Gynecol Neonatal Nurs.* 12(1):21

CHAPTER 6 COMPLICATIONS OF THE ANTEPARTAL PERIOD

INTRODUCTION

A high-risk pregnancy is one in which certain factors or groups of factors increase the possibility of morbidity or even mortality for the mother and/or fetus (or neonate).

This chapter delineates the personal, social, cultural, and environmental factors that might increase the risk. Preexisting conditions, such as maternal heart disease, are then explored, followed by disorders that develop during pregnancy. The final portion of the chapter discusses the infectious processes that may pose a significant threat to maternal, fetal, or neonatal well-being.

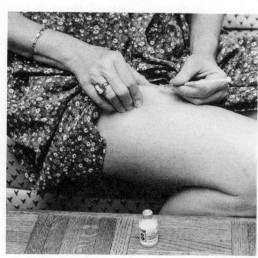

PART I
GENERAL PRINCIPLES AND CONCEPTS

1. What personal characteristics of the mother increase the risk during pregnancy?

   a.

   b.

   c.

   d.

   e.

f.

g.

2. What preexisting medical disorders increase the risk during pregnancy?

a.

b.

c.

d.

e.

f.

g.

3. What obstetric factors present during previous pregnancies increase the risk?

a.

b.

c.

4. What obstetric factors increase the risk for the present pregnancy?

a.

b.

c.

d.

e.

f.

5. What genetic factors increase the risk during pregnancy?

   a.

   b.

Preexisting Conditions

6. Identify three changes that normally occur in the cardiovascular system during pregnancy.

   a.

   b.

   c.

7. The New York Heart Association classification of functional capacity is used to assess the severity of cardiac disease. For each of the classes, state the expected physical activity level.

   a. Class I

   b. Class II

c. Class III

d. Class IV

8. Sandy Jones is a 24-year-old patient who had rheumatic fever as a child and is now considered a class II cardiac patient. List five signs and symptoms that would lead you to suspect cardiac decompensation in Sandy.

a.

b.

c.

d.

e.

9. During the antepartal period, what information would you give Sandy about the following?

a. Nutrition

b. Rest

c. Protection from infection

d. Activity restrictions

e. Frequency of prenatal visits

10. In addition to iron and vitamin supplements, Sandy is started on penicillin prophylaxis. Why is this done?

11. In the absence of complications, what is the method of choice for delivering Sandy's baby?*

12. Compare the signs and symptoms of hyperthyroidism and hypothyroidism in a pregnant woman.

HYPERTHYROIDISM	HYPOTHYROIDISM

13. The main risks for the infant of a hypothyroid mother include

a.

b.

c.

*These questions are addressed at the end of Part I.

Diabetes Mellitus and Pregnancy

14. Define the following as they are used in the classification of diabetes mellitus developed by the National Diabetes Data Group:

    a. Diabetes mellitus

        ● Type I, insulin dependent (IDDM)
        ● Type II, noninsulin-dependent (NIDDM)
        ● Secondary diabetes

    b. Impaired glucose tolerance (IGT)

    c. Gestational diabetes (GDM)

15. Pregnancy has been described as having a diabetogenic effect.

    a. Define the diabetogenic effect of pregnancy.

    b. Identify three physiologic factors that contribute to the diabetogenic effect of pregnancy.

        ●
        ●
        ●

16. Identify five maternal and/or fetal complications that may occur during pregnancy as a result of diabetes mellitus.

    a.

    b.

    c.

    d.

    e.

17. In caring for a pregnant woman with diabetes mellitus, what general information would you give her about the following areas of concern?

   a. Dietary regulation

   b. Urine testing

   c. Insulin requirements

   d. Exercise

   e. Symptoms of hypoglycemia

   f. Frequency of prenatal visits

18. A friend of yours is diagnosed as having gestational diabetes. She tells you that her grandmother takes tolbutamide (Orinase) for her diabetes and asks why she can't simply take tolbutamide too. What would you tell her?*

19. Your friend also asks why infants of diabetic mothers are frequently so large. How would you explain this phenomenon?

*These questions are addressed at the end of Part I.

20. Name three tests that might be performed to assess fetal status in a pregnant patient with diabetes mellitus.

    a.

    b.

    c.

21. Define *hyperemesis gravidarum*.

22. Identify three goals of therapy in treating a patient hospitalized with hyperemesis gravidarum.

    a.

    b.

    c.

Bleeding Disorders

Bleeding at any time during pregnancy is considered a potential problem and requires evaluation. Abortion is the major bleeding disorder associated with the first and second trimesters of pregnancy.

23. Define the following terms:

  a. Abortion

  b. Therapeutic abortion

  c. Spontaneous abortion (miscarriage)

  d. Threatened abortion

  e. Imminent abortion

  f. Complete abortion

  g. Incomplete abortion

h. Missed abortion

i. Habitual abortion

24. Alys Roberts, a 22-year-old gravida I para 0, 11 weeks pregnant, was admitted to the hospital with moderate vaginal bleeding and some abdominal cramping. Vaginal examination reveals that the cervix is dilated 2 cm. She is diagnosed as having an imminent abortion. Identify four nursing interventions that are indicated in caring for Alys.

a.

b.

c.

d.

25. Alys is placed on bedrest with intravenous fluids and that evening passes some of the products of conception. The following morning she has a dilation and curettage (D and C). Why is this done?

26. Alys's husband asks you why abortions occur. Identify four causes of spontaneous abortion.

    a.

    b.

    c.

    d.

27. The most common cause of second trimester abortion is incompetent cervix. Identify two factors that may contribute to incompetent cervix.

    a.

    b.

28. A surgical procedure used to treat incompetent cervix so that a woman may successfully carry a pregnancy to term is _____.

29. Define *ectopic pregnancy*.

30. Identify four possible implantation sites of an ectopic pregnancy.

    a.

    b.

c.

d.

31. What are four clinical signs or symptoms of ectopic pregnancy?

    a.

    b.

    c.

    d.

32. What procedures may be used to diagnose an ectopic pregnancy?

    a.

    b.

    c.

    d.

33. The most significant problem in ectopic pregnancy is _____.

34. Carla Harris is admitted with a diagnosis of hydatidiform mole. Define *hydatidiform mole*.

35. What signs and symptoms might Carla have exhibited that would lead to this diagnosis?

    a.

    b.

    c.

    d.

    e.

36. Following successful removal of the mole, Carla is advised to avoid pregnancy for a year and to return for periodic measurement of hCG levels. What is the rationale for this advice?*

Pregnancy-Induced Hypertension (PIH) (Preeclampsia-Eclampsia)

37. Bettijean Melvins is a 19-year-old primigravida, 34 weeks' gestation, who is having her routine prenatal examination. As part of your assessment, you check her for signs of preeclampsia. List the three cardinal signs of preeclampsia.

    a.

    b.

*These questions are addressed at the end of Part I.

c.

38. Bettijean's baseline blood pressure is 92/64. At what reading would her blood pressure indicate possible preeclampsia?*_____

39. On the following chart, compare the signs and symptoms of mild preeclampsia and severe preeclampsia:

SIGN	MILD PREECLAMPSIA	SEVERE PREECLAMPSIA
Blood pressure		
Weight gain		
Edema		
Proteinuria		
Hyperreflexia		
Headache		
Epigastric pain		
Visual disturbances		

40. What additional symptom characterizes a patient as having eclampsia rather than severe preeclampsia? _____

*These questions are addressed at the end of Part I.

41. Bettijean is hospitalized with severe preeclampsia. Identify five interventions commonly used in caring for a patient with preeclampsia and the rationale for each.

INTERVENTION	RATIONALE

a.

b.

c.

d.

e.

42. In the hospital Bettijean receives magnesium sulfate intravenously. Why?

43. In monitoring Bettijean you are continually alert for signs of magnesium sulfate toxicity. Identify the three main symptoms.

    a.

    b.

    c.

44. The antagonist for magnesium sulfate is _____.

45. A major hemorrhagic complication that may occur in patients with severe preeclampsia is

    _____.

46. Identify four criteria that you can use to evaluate the effectiveness of Bettijean's treatment.*

    a.

    b.

    c.

    d.

*These questions are addressed at the end of Part I.

Infections and Pregnancy

47. Complete the following chart of the infections that may affect pregnancy:

INFECTION	ORGANISM	METHOD OF TRANSFER	IMPLICATIONS FOR MATERNAL/FETAL/NEO-NATAL WELL-BEING	TREATMENT
Toxoplasmosis				
Rubella				
Cytomegalovirus				
Herpes virus type 2				
Syphilis				
Gonorrhea				
Monilial vaginitis				
Chlamydia				

Selected Answers

This section addresses the asterisked questions found in this chapter.

11. Whenever possible, vaginal delivery is performed, using low forceps and a local or regional anesthetic to decrease the stress of the second stage of labor. This procedure also avoids the hazards associated with abdominal surgery for cesarean section.

18. Oral hypoglycemic agents are used in treating certain types of diabetes. However, because they have been linked to fetal abnormalities, they are contraindicated during pregnancy.

36. HCG levels are measured weekly and then monthly to monitor patient status. Elevated hCG titers may indicate the possible development of choriocarcinoma. Birth control, usually using the pill, is necessary, because it would be difficult to tell whether elevated hCG levels were related to pregnancy or to a developing malignancy.

38. Blood pressure of 122/80 indicates possible preeclampsia. An increase of 30 mm Hg systolic and 15 mm Hg diastolic or blood pressure of 140/90 or greater is indicative of possible preeclampsia.

46. Bettijean's treatment can be considered effective if the following criteria have been met:
    a. Continued fetal well-being or delivery of a healthy infant
    b. Normal maternal blood pressure
    c. Absence of proteinuria
    d. Symptoms of preeclampsia/eclampsia controlled or absent
    e. Mother able to resume activities of daily living
    f. Mother able to care for infant (if delivered)

PART II
SELF-ASSESSMENT GUIDE

The following multiple-choice questions will help you assess your knowledge of the content of this chapter. Select the best answer for each of the questions then refer to the end of Part II to check your answers.

1. Which of the following statements about the nutritional needs of pregnant cardiac patients is most accurate?

   a. They require major increases in iron and calories but decreased sodium.
   b. They require increased protein and iron but minimized sodium intake.
   c. They require optimal amounts of all essential vitamins but restricted caloric and iron intake.
   d. They require increased iron, protein, sodium, carboydrates, and fats.

2. Mary Lewis is pregnant for the second time. Her first child weighed 9 lb 11 oz. Her doctors perform a glucose tolerance test and discover elevated blood sugar levels. Because Mary shows no signs of diabetes when she is not pregnant, she is best classified as having

   a. Type I diabetes mellitus.
   b. Type II diabetes mellitus.
   c. Gestational diabetes mellitus.
   d. Secondary diabetes mellitus.

3. In general, patients with Mary's type of diabetes are controlled by

   a. diet therapy.
   b. oral hypoglycemics.
   c. insulin therapy.
   d. all of these.

4. The major cause of spontaneous abortion is

   a. inadequate corpus luteum.
   b. placental inadequacies.
   c. reproductive tract defects.
   d. defects of the ovum or sperm.

5. Tamara Clarkson, at 11 weeks' gestation, calls her doctor and reports that she is having some mild vaginal bleeding and occasional mild cramps but no other problems. She is best characterized as having

   a. a threatened abortion.
   b. a missed abortion.
   c. an imminent abortion.
   d. an incomplete abortion.

6. Which of the following signs would *not* be indicative of a ruptured tubal pregnancy?

   a. Marked lower abdominal pain
   b. Profuse vaginal bleeding
   c. Urinary frequency
   d. Increased pulse and decreased blood pressure

7. Patients with a diagnosis of severe preeclampsia have an increased risk of

   a. complete abortion.
   b. placenta previa.
   c. abruptio placentae.
   d. none of the above.

8. Thrush in the newborn is directly related to contact in the birth canal with which of the following organisms?

   a. *Staphylococcus aureus*
   b. *Neisseria gonorrhoeae*
   c. *Treponema pallidum*
   d. *Candida albicans*

9. In order to protect her unborn child from toxoplasmosis, a pregnant woman should

   a. avoid contact with people known to have German measles.
   b. avoid eating inadequately cooked meat.
   c. avoid sexual relations with known carriers of the causative organism.
   d. be vaccinated against it early in her pregnancy.

10. Which of the following findings would best support a diagnosis of hydatidiform mole?

   a. Elevated hCG levels, enlarged abdomen, absence of quickening
   b. Vaginal bleeding, absence of fetal heart tones, decreased hCG levels
   c. Visible fetal skeleton with sonography, absence of quickening, enlarged abdomen
   d. Brownish vaginal discharge, hyperemesis gravidarum, absence of fetal heart tones

Answers

1. b	6. b
2. c	7. c
3. a	8. d
4. d	9. b
5. a	10. a

SELECTED BIBLIOGRAPHY

Auclair, C.A. January-February 1979. Consequences of prenatal exposure to diethylstilbesterol. *J. Obstet. Gynecol. Neonatal Nurs.* 8:35.

Brown, S.G. May-June 1979. The devastating effects of congenital rubella. *MCN.* 4:171.

Deibel, P. November-December 1980. Effects of cigarette smoking on maternal nutrition and the fetus. *J. Obstet. Gynecol. Neonatal Nurs.* 9:333.

Diabetes in pregnancy. November 1980. *Nurs. 80.* 10:44.

Dore, S.L., and Davies, B.L. March-April 1979. Catharsis for high-risk antepartal inpatients. *MCN.* 4:84.

Federschneider, J.M., et al. April 1980. Natural history of recurrent molar pregnancy. *Obstet. Gynecol.* 55:457.

Fichy, A.M., and Chong, D. March-April 1979. Placental function and its role in toxemia. *MCN.* 4:84.

Gennaro, S. November-December 1980. Listerial infection: nursing care of mother and infant. *MCN.* 5:390.

Good-Anderson, B. March-April 1983. Home blood glucose monitoring in the pregnant diabetic. *J. Obstet. Gynecol. Neonatal Nurs.* 12(2):89.

Gussman, D. November-December 1980. Otosclerosis and pregnancy. *MCN.* 5:408.

Harger, J.H. November 1980. Comparison of success and morbidity in cervical cerclage procedures. *Obstet. Gynecol.* 56:543.

Jones, M.B. March-April 1979. Hypertensive disorders of pregnancy. *J. Obstet. Gynecol. Neonatal Nurs.* 8:92.

Mocarski, V. July-August 1980. Asymptomatic bacteriuria: a "silent" problem of pregnant women. *MCN.* 5:238.

Perley, N.Z., and Bills, B.J. May-June 1983. Herpes genitalis and the childbearing cycle. *MCN.* 8(3):213.

Snyder, D.J. May-June 1979. The high-risk mother viewed in relation to a holistic model of the childbearing experience. *J. Obstet. Gynecol. Neonatal Nurs.* 8:164.

Sonstegard, L. March-April 1979. Pregnancy-induced hypertension: prenatal nursing concerns. *MCN.* 4:90.

Weil, S.G. 1981. The unspoken needs of families during high-risk pregnancies. *Am. J. Nurs.* 81(11):2047.

Willis, S.E. 1982. Hypertension in pregnancy: pathophysiology. *Am. J. Nurs.* 82(5):792.

Willis, S.E., and Sharp, E.S. 1982. Hypertension in pregnancy: prenatal detection and management. *Am. J. Nurs.* 82(5):798.

Werzel, S.K. July-August 1982. Are we ignoring the needs of the woman with a spontaneous abortion? *MCN.* 7(4):258.

CHAPTER 7 *FETAL* ASSESSMENT

INTRODUCTION

A growing body of knowledge about the assessment of fetal status has contributed significantly to the successful outcome of high-risk pregnancies. This chapter considers the most frequently used diagnostic procedures that are currently available.

Procedures that are essentially noninvasive, such as ultrasound and nonstress testing, are presented first. More invasive procedures, such as the oxytocin challenge test and amniocentesis, follow. To provide some practice, sample fetal monitoring strips are provided in the sections on nonstress testing and the oxytocin challenge test.

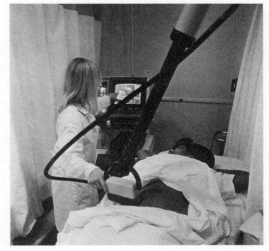

PART I
GENERAL PRINCIPLES AND CONCEPTS

1. List three possible reasons for evaluating fetal status during pregnancy.*

   a.

   b.

   c.

Ultrasound

2. List two advantages for the mother and fetus of using ultrasound for assessment.*

   a.

   b.

*These questions are addressed at the end of Part I.

3. Identify at least six uses of ultrasound during pregnancy.

   a.

   b.

   c.

   d.

   e.

   f.

4. Hazel, gravida II para I, is in her 23rd week of pregnancy. Her last normal menstrual period began 5½ months ago, but she had some bleeding 4½ months ago. Your physical assessment provides the following data: The fundus is palpable at two finger-breadths below the umbilicus; the fetal heart rate (FHR) is 140. Hazel states that she has not felt quickening. Based on this information, why do you think Hazel will have an ultrasound done?

5. Hazel asks you what is involved in having an ultrasound done. How will you respond?

6. When the ultrasound is done, it shows a single fetus with a biparietal diameter (BPD) of 3.5 cm. The fetal heart beat can also be observed.*

    a. Does the BPD correlate with a 20-week-old fetus? _____ If not, what week of gestation is appropriate? _____

    b. What might these results indicate?

7. When BPD is assessed by ultrasound at 40 weeks' gestation, you would expect the diameter to be _____.*

Urinary Estriol

Determination of urinary estriol is a noninvasive method of fetal assessment.

8. List three reasons why urinary estriol may be measured.*

    a.

    b.

    c.

9. What are some implications of a rising level of estriol?

10. What are two implications of a falling estriol level?

    a.

    b.

*These questions are addressed at the end of Part I.

11. How does the administration of ampicillin affect the estriol value?

12. What explanation should the expectant woman receive to ensure correct collection of the urine sample for estriol determination?*

13. What is the critical level (lowest normal value) of estriol at 40 weeks' gestation?* _____

14. If a client has higher than normal estriol levels for her dates, what would you expect the cause to be?*

15. What are the comparative advantages and disadvantages of urinary and plasma estriol determinations?

Nonstress Testing

16. What is the function of a nonstress test (NST)?

17. Explain the procedure for performing an NST.

18. Fetal heart rate patterns in NST have been classified in three ways. What would a fetal monitoring strip show in each case? What further testing may be indicated?

    a. Reactive

    b. Nonreactive

    c. Sinusoidal

19. Label each section of Figure 7-1 as reactive, nonreactive, or sinusoidal.*

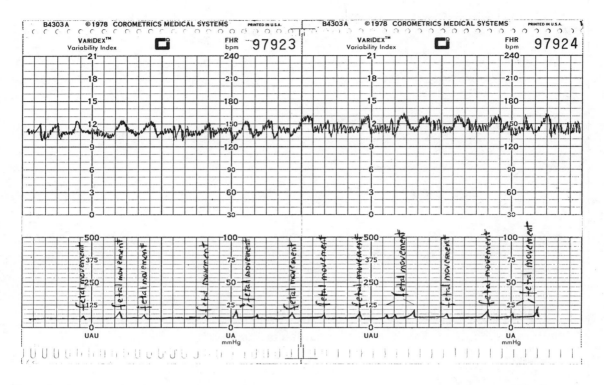

Figure 7-1A. _____

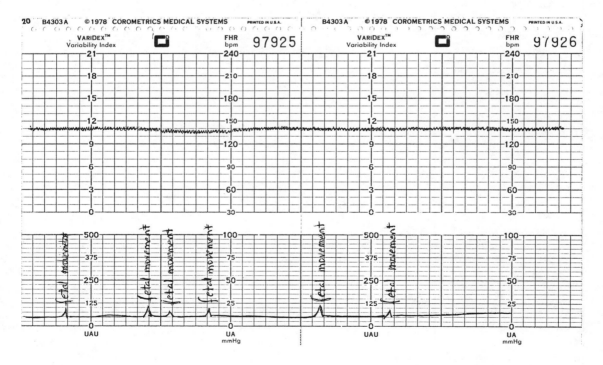

Figure 7-1B. _____

*These questions are addressed at the end of Part I.

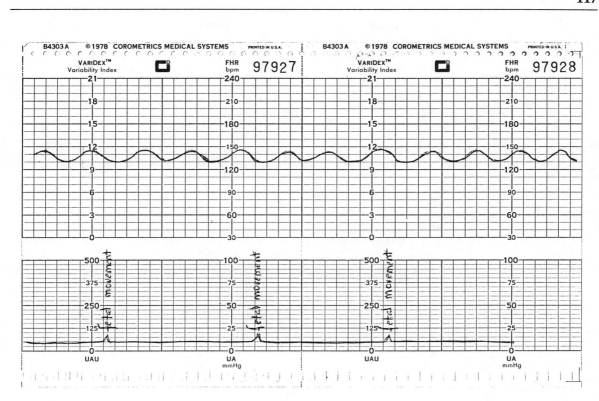

Figure 7-1C. _____

Stress Testing

20. List six indications for doing a contraction stress test (CST). *

  a.

  b.

  c.

  d.

  e.

  f.

*These questions are addressed at the end of Part I.

21. List three contraindications for a CST.*

    a.

    b.

    c.

22. Describe the pattern and significance of fetal CST tracings for both positive and negative results.

RESULT	PATTERN OF CST TRACING	SIGNIFICANCE
Positive		
Negative		

23. Label the two CST tracings in Figure 7-2 as positive or negative.*

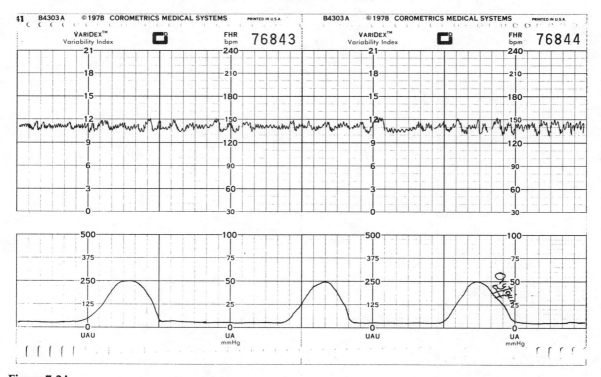

Figure 7-2A. _____

*These questions are addressed at the end of Part I.

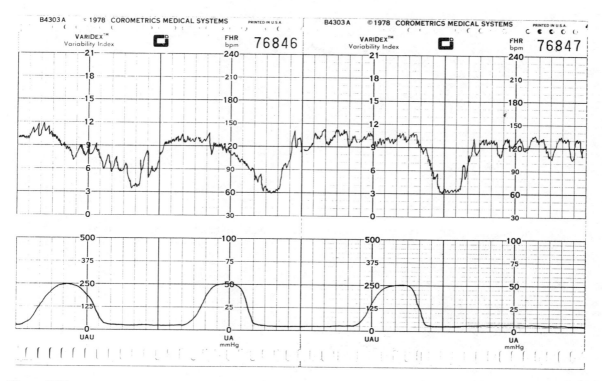

Figure 7-2B. _____

Amniocentesis

24. What is the purpose of amniocentesis?

25. What method may be used to locate the placenta prior to amniocentesis?

26. List three nursing interventions that are necessary during amniocentesis.*

    a.

    b.

    c.

*These questions are addressed at the end of Part I.

27. List three complications associated with amniocentesis.

   a.

   b.

   c.

28. What physical signs and symptoms should a woman be instructed to report after amniocentesis?

29. Identify four tests that may be performed on amniotic fluid.

   a.

   b.

   c.

   d.

30. List three indications for genetic amniocentesis.

   a.

   b.

   c.

31. Identify two conditions that may be associated with abnormalities in chromosome number.

    a.

    b.

32. Identify two conditions that may be associated with abnormalities in sex chromosomes.

    a.

    b.

33. What is the significance of elevated levels of alpha-fetoprotein in the amniotic fluid?

A sample of amniotic fluid may be used to determine the lecithin/sphingomyelin (L/S) ratio.

34. Why is the L/S ratio determined?

35. Adequate levels of lecithin indicate sufficient amounts of pulmonary _____.

36. Fetal lung maturity is attained when the L/S ratio is _____.

A creatinine level may also be determined from an amniotic fluid sample.

37. Why is the creatinine level used as a test of fetal maturity?

38. At 37 weeks' gestation, the normal creatinine level would be _____.

39. Why might elevated creatinine levels appear in the amniotic fluid of a diabetic mother?

Selected Answers

This section addresses the asterisked questions found in this chapter.

1. An evaluation of fetal status may be needed in the presence of any of the following:

    a. failure of the uterus to enlarge at the expected rate or accelerated enlargement.
    b. failure to auscultate fetal heart beat.
    c. medical complications during pregnancy, such as diabetes and preeclampsia-eclampsia.
    d. problems with previous pregnancies, such as fetal death, premature infant, and intrauterine growth retardation (IUGR).

    This list is not all-inclusive but does identify some major factors. If you had difficulty with this question, you should review prenatal complications in your textbook.

2. Some advantages of ultrasound testing are that

    a. it is noninvasive.
    b. it is a painless procedure with the exception of discomfort from a full bladder and from having to lie on one's back for a while.
    c. there is no radiation involved, as with x-rays.
    d. no specific ill effects are now known.
    e. it allows for differentiation of soft tissue.
    f. immediate information can be gained.

6. a. No. It correlates with 17 weeks' gestation.
    b. The results may indicate intrauterine growth retardation or missed dates. In either case, serial ultrasound tests will be done to obtain additional information. If the fetus continues to grow at an appropriate rate, then you may begin to suspect that the menstrual dates were inaccurate. Remember that Hazel said there was some bleeding 4 weeks after her last normal menstrual period. If conception did not occur until after the last "bleeding" episode, then all your information would be off by 3-4 weeks. It's important to identify factors and formulate suspicions, but don't jump to conclusions without sufficient data.

7. At 40 weeks' gestation, the "norm" for BPD is 9.25 cm.

8. Urinary estriol may be used as an assessment method when there are such complications as
    a. preeclampsia-eclampsia.
    b. chronic hypertension.
    c. diabetes.
    d. the possibility of IUGR.

12. The client must receive the following instructions:
    a. Discard the first morning specimen, and then collect all your urine for the next 24 hours.
    b. The urine container must be refrigerated during collection to prevent the formation of bacteria and the breakdown of estrogen products.
    c. As soon as all your urine is collected, it should be taken to the laboratory, so that the test can be run on the same day.
    d. Record any missed (forgotten) voidings, because they may influence the results.

13. At 40 weeks gestation, the critical level of estriol is 12 mg/24 hours.

14. An exceedingly high estriol level may be associated with

    a. a more advanced pregnancy than previously determined.
    b. multiple gestation.
    c. macrosomic fetus (if the mother is diabetic).

19. Figure 7-1A is reactive; B is nonreactive; C is sinusoidal.

20. Indications for a CST include the following:

    a. IUGR
    b. diabetes mellitus
    c. heart disease
    d. preeclampsia-eclampsia
    e. sickle-cell disease
    f. suspected postmaturity
    g. history of previous stillborn
    h. Rh sensitization
    i. abnormal estriol excretion
    j. hyperthyroidism
    k. renal disease

21. Contraindications for a CST include the following:

    a. third-trimester bleeding
    b. previous cesarean birth
    c. instances in which the possible risk of premature labor outweighs the advantages of the CST.

23. Figure 7-2A is a negative CST; B is a positive CST.

26. Nursing interventions during an amniocentesis should include the following:

    a. prepare the equipment.
    b. cleanse the abdomen.
    c. assess the maternal vital signs and the FHR prior to amniocentesis and after the procedure is completed.
    d. document amniocentesis in the client's chart.
    e. provide information and support to the client.

PART II
SELF-ASSESSMENT GUIDE

The following multiple-choice questions will help you assess your knowledge of the content of this chapter. Select the best answer for each of the questions and then refer to the end of Part II to check your answers.

1. An ultrasound reading is done prior to amniocentesis to

    a. avoid any large pockets of amniotic fluid.
    b. decide if the fetus is mature enough.
    c. determine fetal lung maturity.
    d. locate the placenta.

2. Immediately after amniocentesis is completed, the expectant mother complains of dizziness and shortness of breath. Which of the following would best explain the cause?

    a. Pressure of the physician's hands while he or she was withdrawing fluid
    b. Pressure of the uterus on the vena cava while the woman has been lying on her back
    c. The size of the needle that was used
    d. The normal result of having amniotic fluid withdrawn from the uterus

3. A woman calls back 2 hours after having amniocentesis done. She reports that she is having contractions every 5 minutes and is leaking clear fluid. Your best response is that

    a. this is a normal result of amniocentesis.
    b. she should notify her physician and proceed to the labor and delivery unit.
    c. she should rest and call back in 8 hours if the contractions have not subsided.
    d. she should time her contractions for 4 hours and then call the physician.

4. A client has had several diagnostic tests done in the past 2 days. The results are BPD 9.5 cm; creatinine 2 mg/dL; L/S 2.5:1. If she begins labor and delivers today, you know that

   a. she will have a term infant.
   b. she may have twins.
   c. she will have a stillborn fetus.
   d. you should alert a pediatrician and the intensive care nursery to expect a preterm infant.

5. If a client's urinary estriol level falls from 12 mg/24 hours to 4 mg/24 hours, you would suspect

   a. a full-term infant.
   b. a macrosomic infant.
   c. a multiple gestation.
   d. impending fetal death.

6. A CST would most likely be done for a patient who has

   a. a fetal L/S ratio of 1.5:1.
   b. a nonreactive NST.
   c. had amniocentesis for genetic assessment.
   d. had twins.

7. The results of a CST show three contractions in 10 minutes without late decelerations. The CST is

   a. negative.
   b. positive.
   c. suspicious.
   d. unsatisfactory and must be reported.

8. An example of a sex chromosome abnormality is

   a. Down's syndrome.
   b. Tay Sachs disease.
   c. Trisomy 13.
   d. Turner's syndrome.

Answers

1. d 5. d
2. b 6. b
3. b 7. a
4. a 8. d

SELECTED BIBLIOGRAPHY

Afriat, C.I. March-April 1981. The evolution of an antepartum testing program. *J. Obstet. Gynecol. Neonatal Nurs.* 10:110.

Amankwah, K.S., et al. July 1980. A new definition of nonstress test. *Obstet. Gynecol.* 56:48.

Coleman, C.A. January-February 1981. Fetal movement and fetal outcome in a low-risk population. *J. Nurs. Midwifery.* 26:24.

Gibbons, J.M., and Nagle, P. May 1980. Correlation of nonstressed fetal heart rate with sequential contraction stress test. *Obstet. Gynecol.* 55:612.

Johnson, T.R.B., Jr., et al. May 1980. Plasma estriol in the evaluation of third-trimester gestational age. *Obstet. Gynecol.* 55:621.

Kohn, C.L., et al. March-April 1980. Gravidas' responses to realtime ultrasound fetal image. *J. Obstet. Gynecol. Neonatal Nurs.* 9:77.

Lieber, M.T. September-October 1980. "Non stress" antepartal monitoring. *MCN.* 5:335.

Milne, L.S., and Rich, O.J. Spring 1981. Cognitive and affective aspects of the responses of pregnant women to sonography. *Maternal-Child Nurs. J.* 10:15.

O'Brien, G.D. April 1983. Fetal femur—a new dimension of growth. *Contemp. OB/GYN.* 21:186.

Oh, W. April 1983. Heading off problems in the IUGR neonate. *Contemp. OB/GYN.* 21:177.

CHAPTER 8

LABOR
AND DELIVERY:
STAGES AND PROCESSES

INTRODUCTION

Successful labor and delivery results from the effective interplay of anatomic, physiologic, and psychologic factors. These factors, frequently referred to as the "four Ps," include the passage, the passenger, the powers, and the psyche.

This chapter considers the role of each of these factors in the process of birth. It begins with pertinent terminology and focuses on significant aspects of the four Ps. It then focuses on the mechanisms of labor and the stages into which labor and delivery are divided.

Subsequent chapters will relate this basic content to the needs and care of the laboring woman.

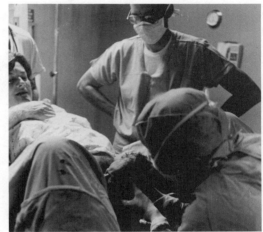

PART I
GENERAL PRINCIPLES AND CONCEPTS

Passage

1. List the four types of pelves, according to the Caldwell-Moloy classification.
   a.

   b.

   c.

   d.

2. Complete the following chart:

PELVIC TYPE	INCI-DENCE	MAJOR CHARACTERISTICS OF:			IMPLICATIONS FOR LABOR AND DELIVERY
		INLET	MIDPELVIS	OUTLET	
Gynecoid					
Android					
Anthropoid					
Platypelloid					

Passenger

3. Label the parts of the fetal skull indicated in Figure 8-1.

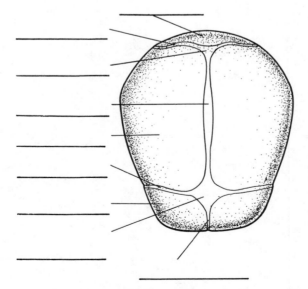

Figure 8-1. Superior view of the fetal skull.

4. Define *suture*.

5. Describe the location of the following:
   a. Mitotic (frontal) suture

   b. Sagittal suture

   c. Coronal suture

   d. Lambdoidal suture

6. Define *fontanelle*.

7. Describe the location and characteristic size of the following:
   a. Anterior fontanelle

   b. Posterior fontanelle

8. Label the landmarks of the fetal skull indicated on Figure 8-2.

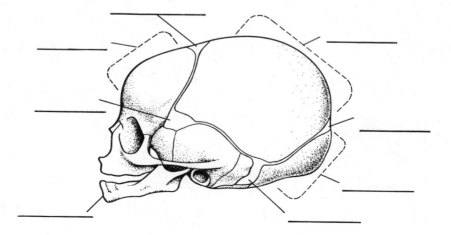

Figure 8-2. Lateral view of the fetal skull.

128

9. Figure 8-3 depicts the anteroposterior and transverse diameters of the fetal head. Label each of the diameters and state their "norms."

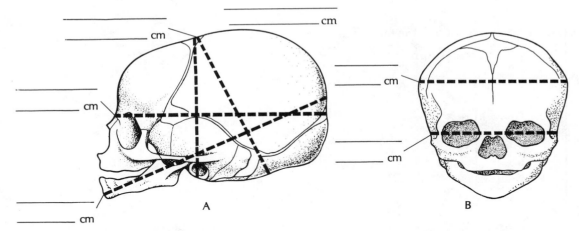

_____
_____ cm
_____ cm
_____
_____ cm
_____ cm

_____
_____ cm

_____
_____ cm

A   B

Figure 8-3. **A**, Anteroposterior diameters of the fetal skull. **B**, Transverse diameters of the fetal skull.

10. Define *fetal attitude*.

11. Define *fetal position*. How does it differ from fetal attitude?

12. Define *fetal lie*.

13. Draw a fetus in a longitudinal lie and a transverse lie on Figure 8-4.

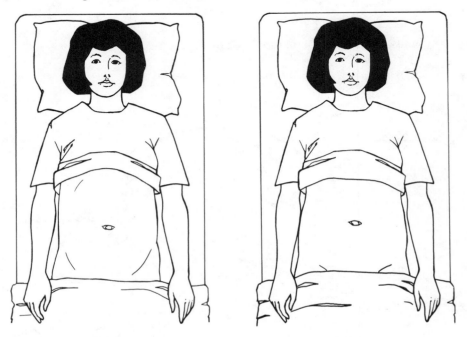

Figure 8-4. Fetal positions. **A**, Longitudinal lie. **B**, Transverse lie.

14. Define *fetal presentation*.

15. List the four types of cephalic presentation.

    a.

    b.

    c.

    d.

16. List and describe the three types of breech presentation.

    a.

    b.

    c.

17. Label the fetal presentations and positions shown in Figure 8-5.*

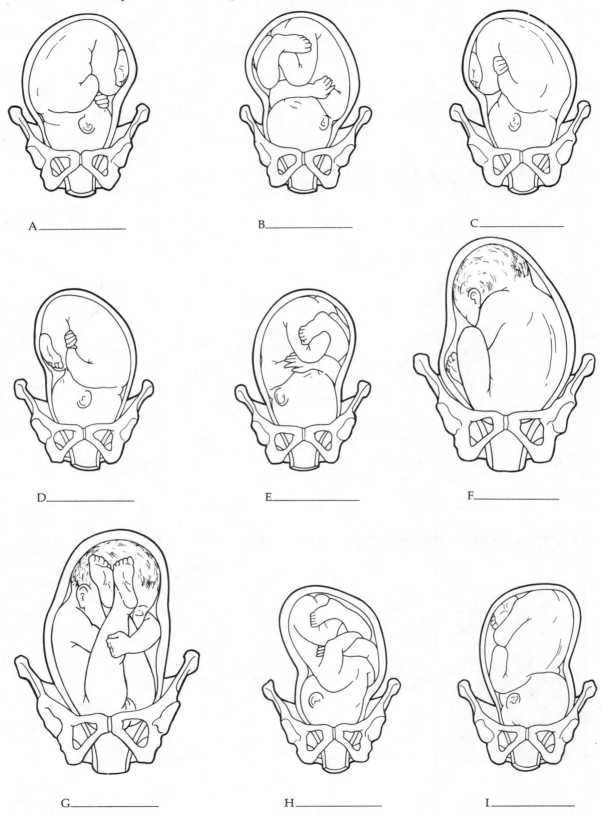

A_____

B_____

C_____

D_____

E_____

F_____

G_____

H_____

I_____

*These questions are addressed at the end of Part I.

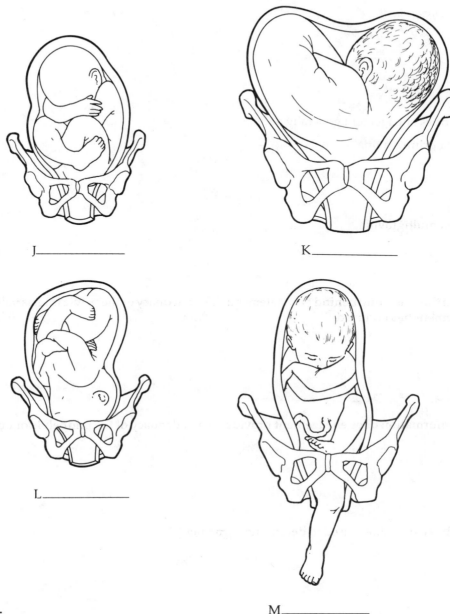

J_____ K_____

L_____

M_____

Figure 8-5.

18. Figure 8-5. List three methods that could be used to determine presentation and position.*

a.

b.

c.

*These questions are addressed at the end of Part I.

19. Define *engagement*.

20. When does engagement generally occur?

    a. For a primigravida

    b. For a multigravida

21. Explain the reasoning behind this statement: "The adequacy of the pelvic inlet is validated once engagement has occurred."*

22. What information does engagement provide about adequacy of the midpelvis or outlet?*

23. Describe two methods used to determine engagment.*

    a.

    b.

24. How would you explain engagement to an expectant mother?

*These questions are addressed at the end of Part I.

25. Devise two questions you could ask the expectant mother that would elicit information about symptoms indicative of engagement. Include your rationale.*

    a.

    b.

26. Define *station*.

27. How is station assessed?

28. Explain what a − 1 station is.

Psyche

29. Identify the factors that may affect a woman's psychologic response to the labor process.

30. Describe how a woman's cultural background might affect her psychologic status in labor.

*These questions are addressed at the end of Part I.

Powers

31. Describe each of the following premonitory signs of labor:

    a. Lightening

    b. Braxton Hicks contractions

    c. Increase in energy

    d. Weight loss

32. The factors that initiate labor are not known, but there are some current theories. Discuss each of the following:

    a. Oxytocin stimulation theory

    b. Progesterone withdrawal theory

    c. Estrogen stimulation theory

    d. Fetal cortisol theory

    e. Fetal membrane phospholipid-arachidonic acid-prostaglandin theory

f. Distention theory

33. Define each of the following terms related to uterine contractions:

a. Increment

b. Acme

c. Decrement

d. Duration

e. Frequency

f. Intensity

34. Label each of the areas indicated in Figure 8-6.

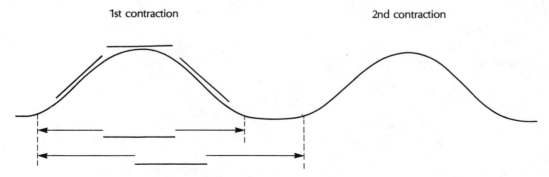

1st contraction   2nd contraction

Figure 8-6. Characteristics of uterine contractions.

35. The positional changes of the fetus during labor are termed *cardinal movements* (or mechanisms of labor). Describe each of the following components of this process:

    a. Descent and engagement

    b. Flexion

    c. Internal rotation

    d. Extension

    e. Restitution and external rotation

    f. Expulsion

36. Labor and delivery is divided into four stages, each with a definite beginning and ending. Complete the following chart:

STAGE	BEGINS	ENDS
First		
Second		
Third		
Fourth		

37. The first stage of labor is divided into which three phases?

a.

b.

c.

38. Complete the following chart:

CHARACTERIS-TICS OF LABOR	FIRST STAGE: LATENT PHASE	FIRST STAGE: ACTIVE PHASE	FIRST STAGE: TRANSITION PHASE	SECOND STAGE	THIRD STAGE
Average duration for primigravida					
Average duration for multigravida					

CHARACTERISTICS OF LABOR	FIRST STAGE: LATENT PHASE	FIRST STAGE: ACTIVE PHASE	FIRST STAGE: TRANSITION PHASE	SECOND STAGE	THIRD STAGE
Frequency of contractions					
Duration of contractions					
Intensity of contractions					
Cervical dilatation					

Selected Answers

This section addresses the asterisked questions found in this chapter.

17. The answers to this question have been provided because some students have difficulty in determining presentation and position.

    a. ROA   f. LSA   k. LAPA
    b. LOP   g. RSA   l. RMA
    c. LOA   h. LMA   m. Single footling
    d. LOT   i. RMP
    e. ROP   j. LSP

    If you had difficulty with this question, refer back to the definitions of presentation and position. It may also help to use a model of a pelvis with a fetus. This is an important concept to grasp, so keep at it.

18. Methods used to determine fetal presentation and position include

   a. Leopold's maneuvers.
   b. visual inspection of the maternal abdomen.
   c. location of the fetal heart tones.
   d. vaginal examination.
   e. assessment of the mother's greatest area of discomfort (for example, a fetus in the posterior position tends to cause more low back pain).
   f. visualization by ultrasound or x-ray.

21. Engagement occurs when the largest diameter of the presenting part has passed through the pelvic inlet. Once this happens, you have established that the pelvic inlet is adequate. Were you able to explain this? If you are having difficulty picturing this, refer to illustrations in your textbook and look at a model of a pelvis with a fetus.

22. None. Engagement provides information about the inlet but not about the midpelvis or outlet. Fetal descent would provide information about the midpelvis and outlet.

23. Leopold's maneuvers and vaginal examinations can be used to determine engagement. X-ray pelvimetry would also provide this information but would not be used solely to determine engagement of the fetal head.

25. The questions should be directed toward changes the mother might feel once engagement has occurred.

   a. "Have you recently noticed a change in the way your clothes fit?" Rationale: As the fetal head drops into the inlet, there may be a change in the shape of the abdomen. It may seem that the baby has dropped down and away from the mother's body. This causes a change in the way her clothes fit.
   b. "Have you recently noticed that you have to urinate more frequently?" Rationale: As the fetus descends into the pelvis, there may be more pressure on the bladder.
   c. "Have you noticed more discomfort in your pelvic area and your thighs?" Rationale: As the fetus descends into the pelvis, there may be more discomfort. There may also be increased pressure from vasocongestion of the areas below the pelvis (that is, the perineum and the lower extremities).
   d. "Have you noticed easier breathing?" Rationale: As the fetus descends into the pelvis, there may be less pressure on the diaphragm.

   Any of these changes may suggest that engagement has occurred, but they are not diagnostic.

PART II
SELF ASSESSMENT GUIDE

The following multiple-choice questions will help you assess your knowledge of the content of this chapter. Select the best answer for each of the questions then refer to the end of Part II to check your answers.

1. A typical gynecoid pelvis would have which of the following characteristics?

   a. Rounded inlet, nonprominent ischial spines, and wide, round pubic arch
   b. Heart-shaped inlet, prominent ischial spines, and narrow, deep pubic arch
   c. Oval outlet, prominent or nonprominent ischial spines, and normal or moderately narrow pubic arch
   d. Transverse oval inlet, prominent or nonprominent ischial spines, and wide pubic arch

2. At term you would expect the suboccipitobregmatic diameter of the fetal head to be approximately

    a. 8 cm.
    b. 9.5 cm.
    c. 11.75 cm.
    d. 13.5 cm.

3. Engagement of the presenting part occurs when the largest diameter of the presenting part

    a. begins to enter the pelvic inlet but can be dislodged with gentle pressure.
    b. is level with the ischial spines.
    c. passes through the pelvic inlet.
    d. passes through the pelvic outlet.

4. A cephalic presentation includes all of the following *except*

    a. brow.
    b. face.
    c. shoulder.
    d. vertex.

5. Which of the following are considered premonitory signs of labor?

    a. Bloody show, desire to bear down
    b. Desire to bear down, increased vaginal secretions
    c. Lightening, increased vaginal secretions
    d. Rupture of membranes, elevated temperature

6. It is often difficult to distinguish true labor from false labor. In false labor,

    a. contractions are of variable frequency and are relieved by walking.
    b. contractions are felt primarily in the lower back.
    c. contractions increase in frequency, duration, and intensity with progressive cervical dilatation.
    d. contractions seem to start in the back and radiate around the abdomen in a girdlelike fashion.

7. To determine frequency, uterine contractions are timed from the

    a. beginning of one contraction to the beginning of the next.
    b. end of one contraction to the beginning of the next.
    c. end of one contraction to the end of the next contraction.
    d. beginning of one contraction to the end of that contraction.

8. There are a variety of theories regarding the cause of labor onset. One possible cause involves

    a. an increase in the amount of circulating progesterone.
    b. a decrease in the amount of circulating estrogen.
    c. production of endogenous oxytocin by the mother's pituitary gland.
    d. inactivation of phospholipase A_2.

9. The fetus adapts to the birth canal by undergoing some positional changes. Which of the following answers best describes the correct sequence?

    a. Descent and flexion, extension, internal rotation, external rotation
    b. Extension, descent and flexion, internal rotation, external rotation
    c. Internal rotation, descent and flexion, extension, external rotation
    d. Descent and flexion, internal rotation, extension, external rotation

10. A number of assessments may be made while performing a vaginal examination during labor. Which of the following is *least* likely to be determined?

    a. Cervical dilatation
    b. Station
    c. Fetal descent
    d. Diagnosis of twins

Answers

1.	a	6.	a
2.	b	7.	a
3.	c	8.	c
4.	c	9.	d
5.	c	10.	d

SELECTED BIBLIOGRAPHY

Bassell, G.M., et al. July 1980. Maternal bearing-down efforts: another fetal risk? *Obstet. Gynecol.* 56:39.

Butani, P., and Hodnett, E. Summer 1980. Mothers' perception of their labor experiences. *Maternal-Child Nurs. J.* 9:73.

Fischer, S.R. January-February 1979. Factors associated with the occurrence of perineal lacerations. *J. Nurs. Midwifery.* 24:18.

Gaziano, E.P., et al. July 1980. FHR variability and other heart observations during second-stage labor, *Obstet Gynecol.* 56:42.

Lynaugh, K.H. July-August 1980. Alternative positions for childbirth, part I: first stage of labor. *J. Nurs. Midwifery.* 25:11.

Lumley, J. Spring 1983. Preschool siblings at birth: short-term effects. *Birth.* 10:11.

McKay, S.R. May 1981. Second-stage labor: has tradition replaced safety? *AJN.* 81:1016.

Nicholson, J., et al. Spring 1983. Outcomes of father involvement in pregnancy and birth. *Birth.* 10:5.

Queenan, J.T., and Queenan, C.N. February 1983. Health care—Chinese style. *Contemp. OB/GYN.* 21:186.

Roberts, J.R. January-February 1979. The effect of maternal position on labor. *J. Nurs. Midwifery.* 24:37.

Schrag, K. November-December 1979. Maintenance of pelvic floor integrity during childbirth. *J. Nurs. Midwifery.* 24:26.

Seitchik, J. December 1980. Measure of contraction strength in labor: area and amplitude. *Am. J. Obstet. Gynecol.* 138:727.

Young, B.K. August 1980. Fetal blood and tissue pH with variable deceleration patterns. *Obstet. Gynecol.* 56:170.

CHAPTER 9 NURSING ASSESSMENT AND CARE OF THE INTRAPARTAL FAMILY

INTRODUCTION

The intrapartal period marks the completion of pregnancy and the beginning of a new life. It is frequently referred to as a crisis; it is certainly a time of stress, as all aspects of the laboring woman—physiologic and psychologic—are affected.

Today, the labor and delivery nurse must have a thorough understanding of the stages and processes of labor and the ability to correlate that knowledge with observable behavior and changes in the laboring woman and those supporting her. In essence, the nurse's understanding of labor and delivery forms the basis for ongoing assessment, intervention, and evaluation of care during labor and delivery.

This chapter puts a heavy emphasis on assessment, anticipated findings and their significance, and appropriate nursing interventions. Questions related to evaluation are also included to provide guidelines for determining the effectiveness of care.

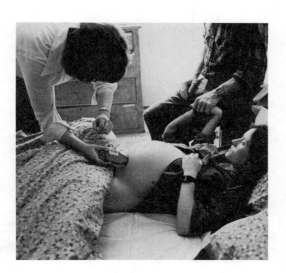

PART I
GENERAL PRINCIPLES AND CONCEPTS

Physical Adaptations to Labor

1. Complete the following chart of maternal and fetal responses to labor:

SYSTEM	EXPECTED CHANGES	PHYSIOLOGIC RATIONALE
Maternal cardiovascular		

SYSTEM	EXPECTED CHANGES	PHYSIOLOGIC RATIONALE
Maternal respiratory		
Maternal renal		
Maternal gastrointestinal		
Maternal hemopoietic		

SYSTEM	EXPECTED CHANGES	PHYSIOLOGIC RATIONALE
Fetal cardiovascular		

Psychosocial Adaptations to Labor

2. Describe the "normal" psychologic response to each phase of the first stage of labor.

   a. Latent phase

   b. Active phase

   c. Transition phase

Clinical Application

3. Adequacy of pelvic diameters should be determined prior to the onset of labor. Complete the following chart:

PELVIC MEASUREMENT	NORMAL RANGE (cm)	ASSESSMENT TECHNIQUE
Diagonal conjugate		
Obstetric conjugate		

PELVIC MEASUREMENT	NORMAL RANGE (cm)	ASSESSMENT TECHNIQUE
True conjugate		
Bituberous width		

4. In Figure 9-1 the solid lines are pelvic diameters and the dotted lines are pelvic planes. Label each of the blanks.

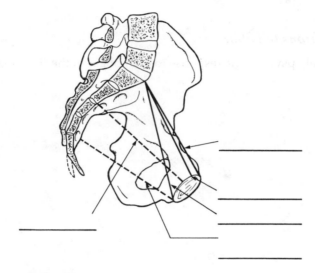

Figure 9-1. Anteroposterior diameters of the pelvic inlet and their relationship to the pelvic planes.

5. The following questionnaire is similar to many that are used when a woman is admitted to the labor and delivery unit. Have a friend or family member act as a patient and role-play a situation in which you, as the labor and delivery nurse, complete the interview. (Note: This questionnaire focuses primarily on baseline information and does not include information that would require physical assessment.)

Admission date: _____ Time: _____

Admitting nurse: _____

Patient name: _____ Age: _____

EDC: _____ LMP: _____ Length of gestation by dates: _____

Attending physician/nurse-midwife _____

Pediatrician: _____

Gravida _____ Para _____ Ab _____ Neonatal deaths _____

Onset of labor: Spontaneous _____ Induced _____ Time _____

Rupture of membranes: Spontaneous _____ Artificial _____ Time _____

Bleeding _____

Blood type _____ Rh _____ Serology _____ Date of serology testing _____

Maternal support: _____ Accompanied by: _____

Prenatal education classes:

Yes _____ No _____ Type _____

Patient requests:

Bottle feeding _____   No anesthesia _____   Rooming in _____

Breastfeeding _____   No medications _____

Father (support person) in delivery room _____

Other _____

Prepregnant weight: _____ Present weight: _____

Medications in current use: _____

Allergies to: Medications _____ Foods _____

Type of food last consumed: _____ Time: _____

Medical problems with this pregnancy: _____

Problems with past pregnancies and labors: _____

Previous illnesses: _____

6. List at least ten intrapartal problems that would contribute to a patient being designated "high risk."*

   a.

   b.

   c.

   d.

   e.

   f.

*These questions are addressed at the end of Part I.

g.

h.

i.

j.

7. Allison Scott is admitted to the labor and delivery department accompanied by her husband, Craig. She is in early labor. During your initial interview, you discover that she is a primigravida and that her EDC is today. She has not attended prenatal classes. What four observations will you make while assessing her contractions?*

a.

b.

c.

d.

8. Why do you use your fingertips instead of the palm of your hand to palpate contractions?

9. What would you expect Allison's contractions to be like if she is in the latent phase?

10. The charge nurse records Allison's contractions as every 5 minutes, lasting 30 seconds, and of mild intensity.

a. What is the frequency? _____   c. What is the intensity? _____

b. What is the duration? _____

*These questions are addressed at the end of Part I.

11. What differences would you perceive when palpating mild, moderate, and strong (intense) contractions?

    a. Mild

    b. Moderate

    c. Strong

12. You will use a fetoscope to assess fetal heart rate (FHR).

    a. Describe the method you will use to locate the FHR.

    b. After locating the fetal heartbeat and just before counting the FHR, you check Allison's radial pulse. Explain the rationale for this.

    c. How long should you listen to the FHR?

13. As part of your assessment, you perform Leopold's maneuvers on Allison. How should she be positioned?*

14. Identify one advantage to performing Leopold's maneuvers prior to locating the FHR.

15. Explain why membrane status should be ascertained before a vaginal examination is done.*

16. What effect do intact membranes have on labor progress?

17. Explain the implications of ruptured membranes for the mother and fetus.

18. Why do you need to know the exact time that the membranes rupture?*

*These questions are addressed at the end of Part I.

19. Explain why the FHR is assessed immediately after the membranes have ruptured.

20. Explain what you will tell the woman if her membranes are ruptured.

21. Allison states that she is losing some clear fluid from her vagina when she coughs. You note that a Nitrazine test tape does not change color.

    a. Are the membranes intact or ruptured?* _____

    b. What do you think the source of the clear fluid is?* _____

22. You do a vaginal examination on Allison.

    a. List the information that can be ascertained by performing a vaginal examination.*

    b. How do you position Allison for the vaginal examination?

    c. Define *cervical dilatation*. How is dilatation recorded?

    d. Define *cervical effacement*. How is effacement recorded?

23. During the vaginal examination you find that you can place two fingers side by side in Allison's cervix. You can feel a firm surface against the cervix and a softer triangular shape in the upper right portion (between 12 and 3 on a clock). You also note a small amount of bloody show.

    a. What is the cervical dilatation?* _____

    b. What is the presentation?* _____

    c. What is the position?* _____

    d. What causes the bloody show?

*These questions are addressed at the end of Part I.

24. List the routine admission laboratory work you would expect to be ordered for Allison.

25. The obstetrician has ordered a "miniprep" and a Fleet's enema for Allison.
    a. Allison does not understand what a "prep" is. How will you explain it to her?

    b. Explain the difference between a "miniprep" and a full prep (according to your agency, as applicable).

    c. What are three reasons for administering an enema?*

    d. What safety factors should you consider when she is ready to expel her enema?*

    e. Explain why the FHR should be taken immediately after the enema is expelled.*

26. Allison will receive only clear liquids or ice chips during labor. Explain the rationale for this.

27. Choose a breathing technique commonly used in your area.
    a. Using it, give Allison a lesson in how to breathe during contractions.

    b. How will this vary during transition?

*These questions are addressed at the end of Part I.

c. Explain the correct procedure for pushing when Allison reaches the second stage.

28. What can you do to help Craig during the labor and delivery process? How can you assist him in supporting Allison?

29. As labor continues, you will use a Friedman graph to chart Allison's progress. Record the following information on Figure 9-2:*

    10 AM, 4 cm, −1
    11 AM, 5 cm, −1
     1 PM, 7 cm,   0
     2 PM, 9 cm, +1
     3 PM, almost complete, +2
     4 PM, complete, +3

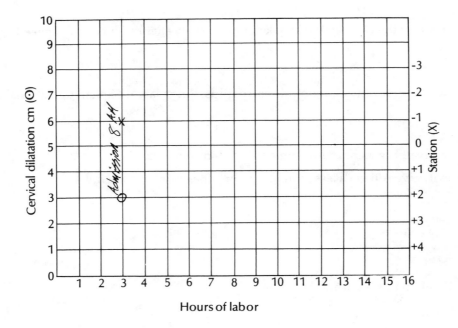

Figure 9-2. Sample Friedman graph. (Modified from Friedman, E. July 1970. An objective method of evaluating labor. *Hospital Practice* 5:87.)

*These questions are addressed at the end of Part I.

30. Allison reaches 7 cm and becomes restless and impatient.

    a. What phase of labor is she in? _____

    b. List nursing interventions that would be useful in helping Allison.

    c. What observations would indicate that your interventions were effective?

31. Allison complains of tingling and numbness in her hands and feet.

    a. What is the cause?*

    b. List nursing interventions to assist Allison.

32. Allison reaches complete dilatation.

    a. Complete dilatation is _____ cm.

    b. What stage of labor is Allison in? _____

33. List signs that indicate delivery is imminent.*

*These questions are addressed at the end of Part I.

154

34. You accompany Allison and Craig to the delivery room. How will you position Allison on the delivery table to facilitate pushing?

35. How often will you need to assess blood pressure and FHR until delivery?

36. Describe the correct procedure for doing a perineal prep prior to delivery (according to your agency's policy).

37. Explain the support measures that you or Craig can use to help Allison feel more comfortable in the delivery room.

38. A midline episiotomy is done. State the reasons for doing an episiotomy.*

*These questions are addressed at the end of Part I.

39. How does a midline episiotomy differ from a mediolateral episiotomy? Complete the following chart:

CHARACTERISTIC	MIDLINE EPISIOTOMY	MEDIOLATERAL EPISIOTOMY
Indication		
Location		
Healing		
Discomfort after delivery		

40. As the baby's head begins to emerge, the obstetrician supports it with his or her hand. Explain the rationale for this.

41. Why is the baby's nose and mouth suctioned as soon as the head has emerged?

42. Allison delivers an infant boy. Your first assessment of him provides the following information:

Heart rate 124
Respirations 24 and irregular
Flexion and movement of all extremities

Vigorous crying when suctioned
Pink body with some acrocyanosis

	0	1	2
Heart rate	Absent	Slow (below 100)	Above 100
Respiratory effort	Absent	Slow, irregular	Good crying
Muscle tone	Flaccid	Some flexion of extremities	Active motion
Reflex irritability	None	Grimace	Vigorous cry
Color	Pale, blue	Body pink, extremities blue	Completely pink

Figure 9-3. Sample Apgar scoring sheet. (Modified from Apgar, V. August 1966. The newborn (Apgar) scoring system: reflection and advice. *Pediatr. Clin. N. Am.* 13:645).

a. Record the above assessments on the Apgar scoring sheet (Figure 9-3).

b. What is the total Apgar score?* _____

c. Apgar scores are assessed at _____ minutes and _____ minutes following delivery.

43. Describe the appearance of a newborn who had an Apgar score between 3 and 6.

44. Summarize the immediate measures that should be initiated for a newborn with an Apgar score of 3-6.

45. Describe the appearance of a newborn who had an Apgar score between 0 and 2.

46. Summarize the immediate measures that should be initiated for the newborn with an Apgar score of 0-2.

*These questions are addressed at the end of Part I.

47. List five major goals of nursing care for the normal newborn.*

    a.

    b.

    c.

    d.

    e.

48. List the methods that may be used to provide warmth to the newborn in the delivery room.

49. Why should the newborn be dried thoroughly as soon after delivery as possible?

50. Allison's newborn is placed under a radiant heater. Explain how the radiant heater works.

51. Why is it necessary to assess the number of vessels in the umbilical cord?

52. How many vessels should there be? _____

*These questions are addressed at the end of Part I.

158

53. List two methods of assuring correct identification of the newborn in the delivery room.*

   a.

   b.

54. In what position is the baby placed to facilitate drainage of the respiratory tract?

55. What complication may result from vigorous, frequent oral suctioning?

56. List the areas that will be checked during a brief physical assessment of the newborn in the delivery room.*

57. Describe methods you can use to facilitate bonding in the delivery room.

58. List specific maternal behaviors that would indicate Allison is beginning to establish bonding.

59. List four signs that indicate separation of the placenta.

   a.

   b.

*These questions are addressed at the end of Part I.

c.

d.

60. Describe differences between a Shultze and a Duncan delivery of the placenta.
    a. Method of separation from the uterine wall

    b. Appearance of placenta at the moment of exit from the vagina

61. Identify the complications that may be associated with a Duncan placenta.

62. List three assessments of the placenta that need to be made following delivery.*

63. The obstetrician orders 10 units of Pitocin given intravenously after delivery of the placenta. Explain the rationale for administration of an oxytocic medication following delivery of the placenta.

64. Compare the oxytocic agents listed in the following chart:

DRUG	DOSE	ROUTE	EFFECT ON UTERUS	SIDE EFFECTS
Pitocin (oxytocin)				
Methergine (methylergonovine maleate)				
Erogotrate (ergonovine maleate)				

*These questions are addressed at the end of Part I.

65. Explain the reason for assessing maternal blood pressure before administering an oxytoxic medication following delivery.

66. You need to record the length of each stage on Allison's delivery record, based on the following information:*

    Contractions began at 8:00 AM
    Complete dilatation at 4 PM
    Delivered male infant at 5:10 PM
    Delivered placenta at 5:25 PM

    a. First stage: _____

    b. Second stage: _____

    c. Third stage: _____

    d. Fourth stage began at _____.

67. How does the length of each of Allison's stages compare with "norms" for primigravidas?

68. Allison is transferred to the obstetric recovery room. List five physical assessments that should be done immediately.*

    a.

    b.

    c.

    d.

    e.

69. Describe the changes you would expect in Allison's vital signs, compared to predelivery levels.

70. What is the significance of a boggy uterus? Describe the immediate action you would take if the uterus was boggy.

71. Allison complains of episiotomy discomfort. List some measures that may alleviate her discomfort.

72. List the data that should be included in your report to the postpartal unit when you transfer Allison from the obstetric recovery room.

73. Karen, a gravida II, para I arrives in active labor and asks to use the birthing room. Describe the following: prenatal preparation that may be needed to use the birthing room; differences in admission process; reasons the use of a birthing room may be denied.

Fetal monitoring is sometimes used during labor.

74. Define the following terms:

    a. Fetal baseline

    b. Fetal tachycardia

    c. Fetal bradycardia

   d. Baseline variability

   e. Early deceleration

   f. Late deceleration

   g. Variable deceleration

75. The normal fetal heart rate is _____ to _____.

76. List five possible causes for fetal tachycardia.*

   a.

   b.

   c.

   d.

   e.

77. List three possible causes for fetal bradycardia.*

   a.

   b.

   c.

*These questions are addressed at the end of Part I.

78. List three possible causes for changes in baseline variability.*
    a.

    b.

    c.

79. Explain the causes of the following:
    a. Early deceleration

    b. Late deceleration

    c. Variable deceleration

80. What findings in FHR tracings would be considered ominous?*

81. Label the fetal monitoring strips shown in Figure 9-4.*

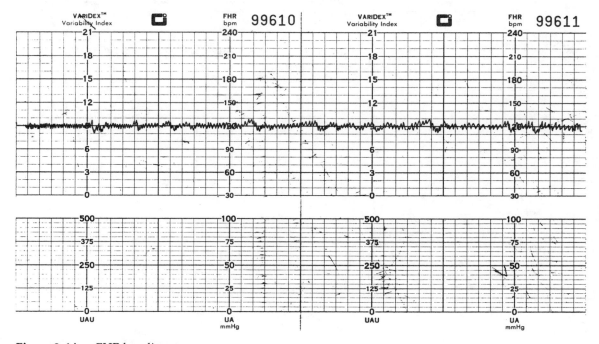

Figure 9-4A. FHR baseline _____

*These questions are addressed at the end of Part I.

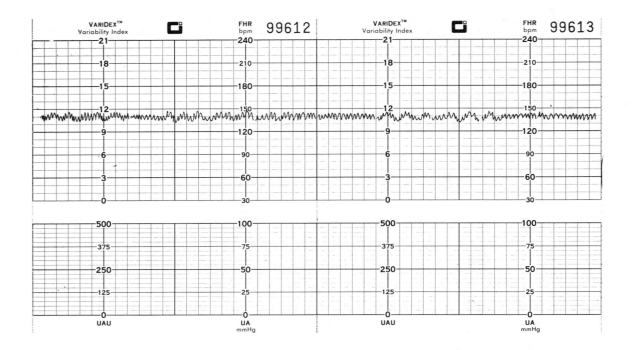

Figure 9-4B. FHR baseline _____

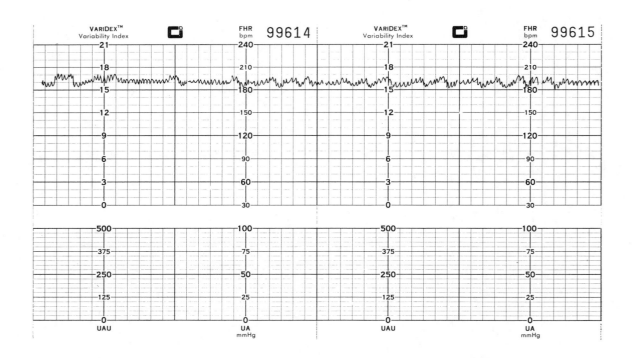

Figure 9-4C. FHR rate _____ ; pattern _____

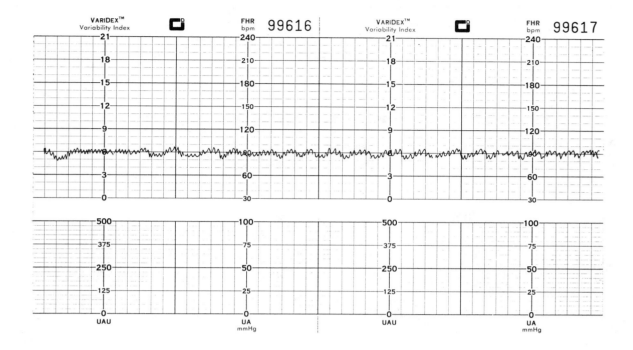

Figure 9-4D. FHR rate _____ ; pattern _____

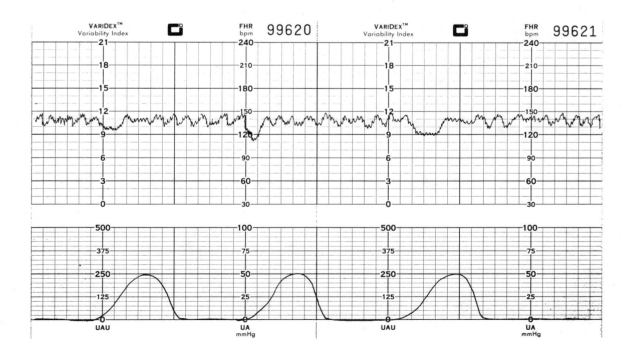

Figure 9-4E. Type of pattern _____

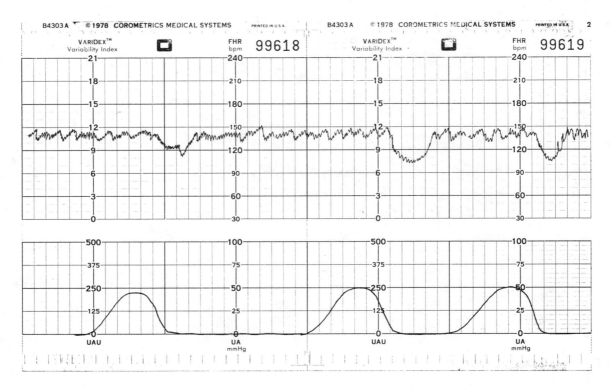

Figure 9-4F.   Type of pattern _____

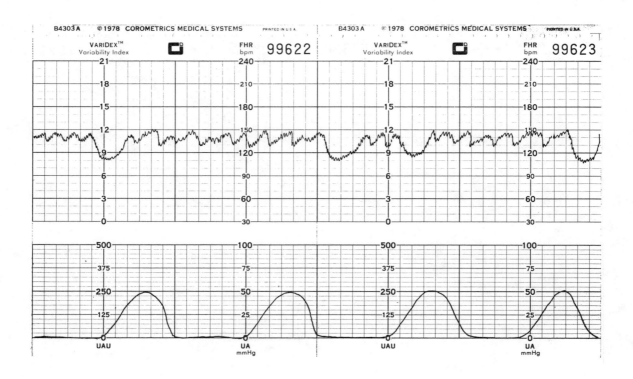

Figure 9-4G.   Type of pattern _____

Induction of Labor

82. List two indications for induction of labor.

    a.

    b.

83. List five contraindications for induction of labor.*

    a.

    b.

    c.

    d.

    e.

Table 9-1.   Prelabor status evaluation scoring (Bishop) system.

| Factor | Assigned value | | | |
	0	1	2	3
Cervical dilatation	Closed	1-2 cm	3-4 cm	5 cm or more
Cervical effacement	0%-30%	40%-50%	60%-70%	80% or more
Fetal station	−3	−2	−1, 0	+ 1 or lower
Cervical consistency	Firm	Moderate	Soft	
Cervical position	Posterior	Midposition	Anterior	

Modified from Bishop, E.H. 1964. Pelvic scoring for elective induction. *Obstet. Gynecol.* 24:266.

84. Explain the Bishop score (see Table 9-1) and the implication of each score for the success of induction.

*These questions are addressed at the end of Part I.

85. Amanda is admitted for a medical induction. She is gravida II, para I, and 42 weeks' gestation. Her membranes are intact. Amanda's obstetrician orders a continuous fetal monitor with a 15-minute baseline, followed by an intravenous induction of 10 units Pitocin in 1000 ml 5% Dextrose in lactated Ringers. The Pitocin is to be started at 1 mU(milliunit)/min by IV infusion pump. How many milliliters per hour will be needed to infuse 1 mU/min?*

86. Five percent Dextrose in water is not routinely used for Pitocin induction because of the risk of water intoxication. Describe the signs of water intoxication.

87. List the physical assessments that must be made prior to increasing Amanda's infusion rate.*

88. List the assessments that would indicate a problem in response to the induction.*

89. After the induction has been in process for 2 hours, you palpate strong contractions and note the following information on the fetal monitoring strip (see Figure 9-5):*

    a. FHR baseline is _____.

    b. Variability is _____.

    c. Contraction frequency is _____.

    d. Contraction duration is _____.

    e. Based on your assessment, should the IV Pitocin infusion rate be advanced? _____

90. After an additional 1 hour of induction, you observe the fetal monitoring strip in Figure 9-6.*

*These questions are addressed at the end of Part I.

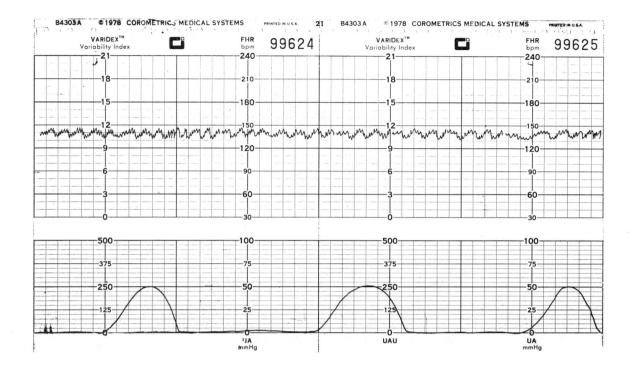

Figure 9-5. Fetal heart rate tracings. Paper speed 3 cm/minute; 6 small spaces equal 1 minute.

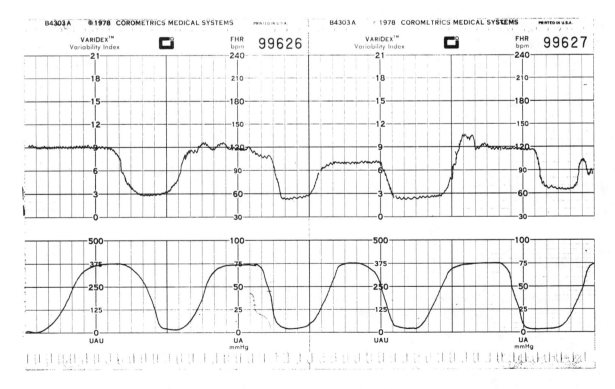

Figure 9-6. Fetal monitoring strip. Paper speed 3 cm/minute; 6 small spaces equal 1 minute.

a. What immediate nursing actions need to be taken?

b. What information from the strip did you use to determine your nursing actions?

91. The obstetrician decides to rupture Amanda's membranes.
    a. Why might this be done?

    b. What two assessments should be made immediately after the membranes are ruptured?*

92. Explain the significance of the following characteristics of amniotic fluid:
    a. Greenish color

    b. Reddish color

    c. Foul odor

Cesarean Birth

93. Janel, gravida II, para I, 39 weeks' gestation, is admitted to labor and delivery for a repeat cesarean section. Her primary section was done for cephalopelvic disproportion (CPD). The L/S ratio is 2.5:1. What instructions would you give Janel in regard to the following?
    a. Abdominal and perineal prep

*These questions are addressed at the end of Part I.

b. Foley catheter

c. Preoperative teaching*

94. Describe the following types of cesarean uterine incisions:
   a. Low segment transverse

   b. Classic

95. List the advantages of a low segment transverse uterine incision.

96. Identify the possible neonatal respiratory complication associated with cesarean birth.*

97. Describe the cause of neonatal respiratory complications associated with cesarean birth.

*These questions are addressed at the end of Part I.

98. Develop a plan of care for Janel in the recovery room.*

PROBLEM	NURSING INTERVENTION	RATIONALE

Evaluation:

99. Explain the possible psychologic reactions to a cesarean delivery.

100. Describe the role of the father during a scheduled cesarean delivery.

Selected Answers

This section addresses the asterisked questions found in this chapter.

6. There are many possible answers to this question. Various authorities have identified intrapartal problems that would contribute to a patient being designated "high risk." Hobel (1976) classifies intrapartal problems as early, interim, and late and assigns a numerical value to each problem. Hobel's list includes

premature labor	pitocin augmentation
hydramnios	prolapse of cord
multiple pregnancy	uterine bleeding
abnormal presentations	FHR deviations
preeclampsia	amnionitis
premature rupture of membranes	excessive maternal medication
cesarean section	maternal seizures
meconium staining of amniotic fluid	forceps delivery
dysfunctional labor	

You should have been able to identify at least ten of these factors. See Hobel, C. 1976. Problem-oriented risk assessment during labor. *Contemporary OB/GYN.* 8:120.

7. There are four pertinent assessments of uterine contractions: intensity, frequency, duration, and the woman's response to the contractions.

13. The woman should be lying on her back with a small pillow under her head. The knees are drawn up, with feet flat on the bed to increase relaxation of the abdominal muscles.

15. The membrane status is ascertained beforehand because the lubricant used for the vaginal examination can change the reactivity of the Nitrazine test tape and thereby give a false reading.

18. Most sources recommend that the woman deliver within 24 hours after rupture of membranes because after that time the incidence of infection increases. You will need to know when they rupture to be able to keep track of the 24 hours.

21. a. The membranes are intact. The Nitrazine test is negative.
    b. The most likely source of the clear fluid is the bladder.

22. a. A number of assessments are made while performing a vaginal examination. You can determine cervical effacement and dilatation; fetal descent, station, position, and presentation; and can assess pelvic measurements.

23. a. 3 cm. If you did not answer this correctly, refer to a cervical dilatation guide in your textbook.
   b. Cephalic. The head feels firm compared to the softer tissues of its buttocks when the fetus is in a breech presentation.
   c. Left-occiput-anterior (LOA). The triangular shape is the posterior fontanelle. If it is felt in the upper portion of the cervix, the fetus is LOA. Refer to Figure 8-5 (or your textbook) for help in visualizing this fetal position. If you answered this question correctly, then you have a good understanding of fetal position.

25. c. Three reasons for administering an enema are to cleanse the lower bowel, to stimulate uterine contractions, and to avoid embarrassment during the second stage of labor.
   d. If the membranes have ruptured, she should expel her enema into a bedpan.
      Consider leaving the siderails up to provide something for her to hold on to. If her labor is advancing rapidly, you will need to assess her labor status frequently. And when she is expelling an enema in the bathroom, she will need to know how to call for assistance.
   e. Auscultation of the FHR will provide information regarding fetal status.

29. A filled-in version of Figure 9-2:

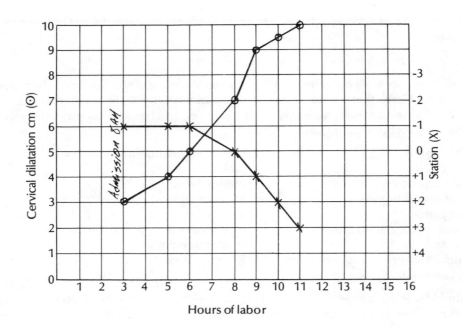

31. a. The cause is hyperventilation, which leads to respiratory alkalosis.

33. The signs that indicate delivery is imminent include a bulging perineum, increased bloody show, +3 station, gaping of the vagina, and an urge to push.

38. An episiotomy is done to prevent excessive stretching of the tissues and to prevent tearing or lacerations of the vaginal and perineal tissues.

42. b. The Apgar score is 8. One point off for respiratory effort and one point off for color.

47. The major goals of nursing care for the newborn include

   a. facilitating respirations.
   b. maintaining temperature.
   c. preventing infection.
   d. providing correct identification.
   e. promoting bonding.

53. a. Application of name bands
    b. Footprinting

56. The brief physical assessment of the newborn should include

    a. overall size and general appearance.
    b. posture and movements.
    c. rate and irregularities of the apical pulse.
    d. respirations (rate, presence of retractions, grunting).

    If the newborn is stable, you may continue by assessing

    e. the head (general appearance, discoloration, fontanelles, flaring of nostrils, condition of palate).
    f. the neck (webbing or any limitation of movement).
    g. the abdomen (size, shape, contour, abnormal pulsations, number of vessels in umbilical cord).
    h. extremities (asymmetry, movement, number of digits).
    i. skin (discolorations, edema).
    j. elimination (record on newborn record any voiding or stools).

62. Assessment of the placenta should include

    a. examination of membranes: a missing section may indicate retention of a piece of membrane in the uterus, and vessels traversing the membranes may indicate placenta succenturiate.
    b. inspection of the umbilical cord for number of vessels, insertion site, and abnormalities, such as knots.
    c. inspection of the placenta for missing cotyledons, infarcts and/or areas of calcification, and overall size and weight.

66. a. First stage: 8 hours
    b. Second stage: 1 hour 10 minutes
    c. Third stage: 15 minutes
    d. Fourth stage: began at 5:25 PM and lasted until 7:25 or 9:25 (2-4 hours)

    If you missed this question, you need to review the definitions of each stage.

68. Immediate physical assessments must include

    a. vital signs (blood pressure, temperature, pulse, respiration)
    b. fundal check (consistency, height, position).
    c. lochia (amount, presence of clots).
    d. perineum (episiotomy, lacerations, bruising, excessive swelling, hemorrhoids).
    e. bladder (distention).

76. The possible causes of fetal tachycardia include

    a. prematurity
    b. mild or chronic fetal hypoxia
    c. fetal infection
    d. frequent repetitive fetal movements
    e. maternal anxiety
    f. maternal drugs
    g. high maternal temperature
    h. fetal arrhythmias (this is uncommon)

77. The possible causes of fetal bradycardia include

    a. fetal hypoxia
    b. sudden hypoxemia
    c. arrhythmia, such as congenital heart block
    d. hypothermia
    e. drugs, such as beta-adrenergic blocking agents (anesthetic agent used for paracervical block)

78. The possible causes for changes in baseline variability include the following:

   a. maternal medications
   b. fetal rest
   c. gestation of less than 32 weeks
   d. fetal hypoxia and acidosis
   e. fetal malformation

80. Ominous findings would be any of the following:

   a. late deceleration
   b. severe variable deceleration
   c. rising FHR baseline
   d. decreasing variability
   e. a slow return to baseline following contractions

81. The fetal monitoring strips depict

   a. FHR baseline of 120.
   b. FHR baseline of 140.
   c. Fetal heart rate 190; fetal tachycardia.
   d. Fetal heart rate 90; fetal bradycardia.
   e. Early deceleration.
   f. Late deceleration.
   g. Variable deceleration.

83. Induction of labor is contraindicated in the presence of any of the following:

   a. cephalopelvic disproportion (CPD)
   b. previous cesarean section for CPD
   c. previous uterine surgery
   d. severe fetal distress
   e. placenta previa
   f. severe or complete abruptio placentae
   g. invasive carcinoma of the cervix
   h. soft tissue masses of reproductive organs or reproductive tract
   i. lack of client acceptance
   j. herpesvirus type 2

   Can you determine why each of these factors would be a contraindication for induction? Many of them are addressed in Chapter 11.

85. The correct answer is 6 mL/hour. To compute this problem, you need to start with the following facts:

   1mL Pitocin = 10 units
   1 unit = 1000 mU (milliunits)
   10 units = 10,000 mU

   $$\frac{10{,}000 \text{ mU}}{1{,}000 \text{ mL}} = \frac{x}{1 \text{ mL}}$$

   $x = 10$ mU/mL of intravenous fluid

   There are 60 minutes in an hour, and you want 1 mU/minute; 60 min $\times$ 1 mU/min = 60 mU/hr

To obtain milliliters per hour:
$$\frac{10\ mU}{1\ mL} = \frac{60\ mU}{x\ mL}$$

$$10\,x = 60$$
$$x = 6\ mL/hr$$

Did you arrive at the correct answer? This problem requires a lot of thought, but it is important to be able to calculate Pitocin infusion rates so that the patient's safety can be maintained.

87. Immediately prior to increasing the rate of intravenous Pitocin infusion, you must assess the following:

   a. maternal blood pressure and pulse
   b. uterine contractions (frequency, duration, intensity)
   c. FHR (rate, response to contraction, variability, reactivity)
   d. fetal response (excessive or cessation of activity)

88. The problems that might occur in response to a Pitocin induction include

   a. tetanic contractions.
   b. late or variable decelerations in FHR.
   c. a significant increase or decrease in maternal blood pressure or pulse.
   d. signs of water intoxication if an electrolyte-free solution is used.

89. The sample fetal monitoring strip provides the following information:

   a. The FHR baseline is 140 for the 8-minute segment. It is best to assess a 10-minute segment to accurately determine the baseline. If you caught this point, congratulations. You had to know the definition of an FHR baseline and correctly count the spaces to realize that only 8 minutes are depicted.
   b. The variability is moderate.
   c. The contraction frequency is every 3 minutes.
   d. The contraction duration is 60-75 seconds.
   e. No. The infusion rate should not be advanced, because "good" contractions have been achieved.

90. The strip indicates severe problems.

   a. The immediate nursing actions would include discontinuing the Pitocin infusion and turning on the main intravenous line; turning the mother on her left side; starting oxygen administration at 4-7 L per minute; notifying the physician; anticipating preparations for effecting an immediate delivery.
   b. The strip showed severe late decelerations with minimal variability and tetanic contractions every 1½ minutes lasting 80–90 seconds.

If you were able to answer this question correctly, you have successfully correlated a lot of information. If you missed it, don't despair. Refer back to your textbook.

91. b. First, the FHR should be assessed immediately after the membranes have been ruptured. The rationale for this action is that the umbilical cord may wash down through the cervix as the amniotic fluid escapes. As pressure is exerted on the cord, the fetal blood supply may be comprised. Second, you need to assess the amniotic fluid for amount, color, and odor.

93. c. The preoperative teaching should include the following information:

   explanation of recovery room and operating room
   turn, cough, and deep breathing routine
   intravenous fluids following surgery

indwelling catheter to drain the bladder
pain relief measures
ambulation following surgery
dietary and fluid restrictions following surgery
nursing assessments that will be done following surgery (vital signs, incisional check, lochia)

96. Wet lung is a possible complication of a cesarean birth.

98. The immediate problems that need to be addressed include the following:

   a. recovery from anesthesia
   b. maintenance of fluids
   c. blood loss
   d. bladder drainage
   e. nausea and vomiting
   f. pain
   g. healing of incision
   h. bowel function

PART II
SELF-ASSESSMENT GUIDE

The following multiple-choice questions will help you assess your knowledge of the content of this chapter. Select the best answer for each of the questions and then refer to the end of Part II to check you answers.

1. You are performing Leopold's maneuvers and determine that the fetus is ROA. Which of the following did you find?

   a. Round, firm object low in pelvis, small parts on mother's right side, and soft rounded shape in fundus
   b. Round, firm object low in pelvis, small parts on mother's left side, and soft rounded shape in fundus
   c. Soft rounded shape in lower pelvis, small parts on mother's right side, and firm, round object in fundus
   d. Soft rounded shape on mother's right side, firm rounded shape on mother's left side, and small parts at the level of the umbilicus

2. Which of the following describes contractions with a frequency of 3 minutes?

   a. A contraction that lasts for 3 minutes, followed by a period of relaxation
   b. Contractions that last for 60 seconds, with a 1-minute rest between contractions
   c. Contractions that last for 30 seconds, with a 2½-minute rest between contractions
   d. Contractions that last for 45 seconds, with a 3-minute rest between contractions

3. You are palpating a uterine contraction and note that during acme the uterine wall cannot be indented with your fingertips. The intensity of the contraction is

   a. mild.   c. intense.
   b. moderate.   d. irregular.

4. You auscultate the FHR and determine a rate of 152. Which of the following actions is appropriate?

   a. Inform the woman that the rate is normal.
   b. Reassess the FHR in 5 minutes, because the rate is too high.
   c. Report the FHR to the physician immediately.
   d. Tell the woman that she is going to have a boy, because the heart rate is fast.

5. While performing a vaginal examination, you determine that the fetus is a cephalic presentation and that the occiput has reached the ischial spines. The station is

   a. −2
   b. −1
   c. 0
   d. +1

6. You note persistent early decelerations on a fetal monitoring strip. Based on your knowledge of this pattern, you would

   a. do nothing. The pattern is benign.
   b. perform a vaginal examination to assess dilatation and to determine whether the mother is ready to push.
   c. stay with the woman and observe what happens during the next contraction.
   d. turn the woman to her left side and start to administer oxygen by mask.

7. A laboring client's membranes rupture suddenly at the end of a contraction. Your first nursing action would be to

   a. assess FHR.
   b. change the bed to enhance the woman's comfort.
   c. instruct the woman to push.
   d. notify the physician immediately.

8. Which of the following women would you expect to have the most rapid labor?

   a. Gravida V, para I, ab III, at term
   b. Gravida II, para I, with breech presentation, at term
   c. Gravida II, para I, with left-occiput-posterior, at term
   d. Gravida II, para I, at 35 weeks' gestation

9. Which of the following would you normally expect if a primigravida with a breech presentation is in the transitional phase of labor?

   a. A decrease in maternal blood pressure
   b. An excessive amount of bloody show
   c. Severe back pain
   d. Slower progress than if the fetus was a vertex presentation

10. You would expect a cesarean delivery for which of the following women?

    a. A gravida II, para I who is dilated 6 cm after 3 hours of labor
    b. A primigravida who is dilated 6 cm after 8 hours of labor and is crying with contractions
    c. A primigravida whose pelvic measurements are diagonal conjugate 12.5 cm, biishial diameter 8.5 cm
    d. A primigravida whose fetal monitoring strip shows an FHR of 60 with contractions and who is dilated 5 cm

11. A multipara who has been in labor for 2 hours suddenly calls for the nurse and says "The baby is coming." After a quick assessment, you determine that the baby will be born with the next contraction. Which of the following interventions should be first?

    a. Call for assistance so the nursery can be notified.
    b. Instruct the woman to pant while you prepare to support the baby's head as it is born.
    c. Instruct the woman to push while you get a clean towel to place under her hips.
    d. Quickly return to the nurse's station to call for a physician.

Answers

1. b	7. a
2. c	8. d
3. c	9. d
4. a	10. d
5. c	11. b
6. a	

SELECTED BIBLIOGRAPHY

Beck, C.T. November-December 1980. Patient acceptance of fetal monitoring as a helpful tool. *J. Obstet. Gynecol. Neonatal Nurs.* 9:350.

Becker, C.H. November-December 1982. Comprehensive assessment of the healthy gravida. *J. Obstet. Gynecol. Neonat. Nurs.* 11:375.

Blair, C., and Mahoukis, C. March-April 1980. Comparing notes: the nurse as patient/the nurse as labor coach. *MCN.* 5:102.

Boyd, S.T., and Mahon, P. May -June 1980. The family-centered cesarean delivery. *MCN.* 5:176.

Britton, G.R. March-April 1980. Early mother-infant contact and infant temperature stabilization. *J. Obstet. Gynecol. Neonatal Nurs.* 9:84.

Burchell, R.C., and Gunn, J. July-August 1980. The new birth experience. *J. Obstet. Gynecol. Neonatal Nurs.* 9:250.

Cranston, C.S. November-December 1980. Obstetrical nurses' attitudes toward fetal monitoring. *J. Obstet. Gynecol. Neonatal Nurs.* 9:344.

Harr, B.D., and Hastings, J.M. January-February 1981. Parturition care planning. *J. Obstet. Gynecol. Neonatal Nurs.* 10:54.

Hart, G. July-August 1980. Maternal attitudes in prepared and unprepared cesarean deliveries. *J. Obstet. Gynecol. Neonatal Nurs.* 9:243.

Lumley, J. Fall 1982. The irresistible rise of electronic fetal monitoring. *Birth.* 9:150.

Maloni, J.A. September-October 1980. The birthing room: some insights into parents' experiences. *MCN.* 5:314.

McDonough, M. January-February 1981. Parents' responses to fetal monitoring. *MCN.* 6:32.

McKay, S.R. September-October 1980. Maternal position during labor and birth: a reassessment. *J. Obstet. Gynecol. Neonatal Nurs.* 9:288.

Meissner, J.E. July 1980. Predicting a patient's anxiety level during labor: a two-part assessment tool. *Nurs. '80.* 10:50.

Norr, K.L., et al. January-February 1980. The second time around: parity and birth experience. *J. Obstet. Gynecol. Neonatal Nurs.* 9:30.

Roberts, J.E. January-February 1979. Maternal positions for childbirth: a historical review of nursing care practices. *J. Obstet. Gynecol. Neonatal Nurs.* 8:24.

CHAPTER 10 *PAIN RELIEF:*
OBSTETRIC ANALGESIA
AND ANESTHESIA

INTRODUCTION

Pain relief during labor and delivery is a subject marked by varying opinions, differences in regional practices, and changing trends. In recent years there has been increased emphasis on teaching expectant families to cope with childbirth so as to decrease or even eliminate the need for medication. Comfort and support measures that the nurse or coach can use to assist the laboring woman have also received renewed attention.

This chapter first explores "nonmedication" approaches to alleviating discomfort and then considers the more traditional analgesics that may be used. Regional and general anesthesia have a significant role in obstetrics, and the chapter concludes with questions about their use and the implications for the mother and fetus.

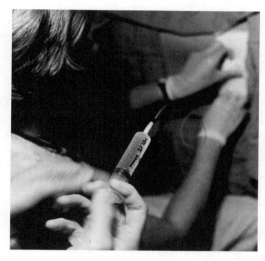

PART I
GENERAL PRINCIPLES AND CONCEPTS

1. List the physiologic factors that contribute to discomfort in each stage of labor.*

    a. First stage

    b. Second stage

    c. Third stage

*These questions are addressed at the end of Part I.

182

2. How do each of the following factors influence the perception of pain in the laboring woman?

   a. Cultural background

   b. Fatigue

   c. Anxiety

   d. Previous experience

3. List three methods that you can teach the laboring woman to help relieve her discomfort during the first stage of labor.*

4. Complete the following chart on analgesic agents commonly used during labor:

*These questions are addressed at the end of part I.

ANALGESIC AGENT	WHEN ADMINISTERED	DESIRED EFFECT	NURSING ACTIONS	SIDE EFFECTS (MATERNAL AND FETAL)
a. Secobarbital sodium (Seconal)				
b. Meperidine hydrochloride (Demerol)				
c. Promethazine (Phenergan)				
d. [†]				
e. [†]				

[†]Include any analgesics commonly used in your area.

5. Barbara Adams, gravida I, para 0, is in the active phase of labor. Contractions are every 3 minutes, lasting 50 seconds, and are moderate. She is 7 cm dilated, 75% effaced, and at 0 station. Her membranes are intact, and the FHR is 140. With each contraction, Barbara cries out and thrashes in the bed. Her restlessness continues between contractions. She repeatedly changes positions and rolls her head from side to side. Her blood pressure and pulse rate have increased over the past 2 hours. The physician has ordered 75 mg of meperidine and 25 mg of promethazine, given intramuscularly when needed for pain. Record at least five actions that you or a support person can use to relieve Barbara's discomfort and the rationale for each.

ACTION	RATIONALE
a.	
b.	
c.	
d.	
e.	

6. How will you evaluate the effectiveness of your actions?

7. If Barbara continues to experience discomfort and needs additional pain relief, what types of regional anesthesia might be given?*

   a. In active labor

*These questions are addressed at the end of Part I.

b. In the second stage

8. Complete the following chart of the regional anesthetic blocks commonly used during labor:

REGIONAL ANESTHETIC BLOCK	USES	NURSING IMPLICATIONS	SIDE EFFECTS (MATERNAL AND FETAL)
Pudendal			
Paracervical			
Epidural			
Spinal			

9. The following chart lists some side effects that may be encountered with the use of regional anesthetic agents. List the appropriate nursing actions for each side effect and explain the rationale.

SIDE EFFECT	INTERVENTIONS	RATIONALE
Hypotension		
Fetal bradycardia		
Uterine inertia		
Bladder distention		

10. General anesthesia is used in most emergency cesarean births and is still used in some regions of the country for normal labor and delivery patients. Nurses must therefore be familiar with commonly used anesthetic agents. Complete the following chart:

ANESTHETIC AGENT	USES	NURSING IMPLICATIONS	SIDE EFFECTS (MATERNAL AND FETAL)
Halothane (Fluothane)			
Ketamine			
Nitrous oxide			

ANESTHETIC AGENT	USES	NURSING IMPLICATIONS	SIDE EFFECTS (MATERNAL AND FETAL)
Methoxy-flurane (Penthrane)			
Thiopental sodium (Pentothal			

Selected Answers

This section addresses the asterisked questions found in this chapter.

1. a. First stage: hypoxia of uterine muscle cells during contractions, stretching of the lower uterine segment and cervix, dilatation of the cervix, and pressure on adjacent structures
   b. Second stage: hypoxia of contracting uterine muscle cells, distention of the vagina and perineum, and pressure on adjacent structures
   c. Third stage: uterine contractions and cervical dilatation as the placenta is expelled

3. Teaching measures to relieve discomfort during the first stage should begin with admission. If you explain what you are going to do before each procedure, the woman will be more comfortable and less anxious. Breathing techniques may be taught during early labor if the mother has not attended prenatal classes. Relaxation techniques and tips are also helpful to relieve discomfort. The woman may be taught to focus on an object during contractions to increase relaxation and comfort. Effleurage may also be helpful.

7. a. In the transition stage, the physician may administer a paracervical, epidural, or caudal block.
   b. In the second stage, the physician may administer a saddle, caudal, pudendal, or local anesthetic.

PART II
SELF-ASSESSMENT GUIDE

The following multiple-choice questions will help you assess your knowledge of the content of this chapter. Select the best answer for each of the questions and then refer to the end of Part II to check your answers.

1. Barbara, a 15-year-old primigravida, is in active labor. She has had no prenatal education. On admission, she asked numerous questions and seemed to become increasingly upset as you explained what the labor and delivery would be like. As labor progresses, she becomes increasingly tense and is not tolerating labor well. You know her level of discomfort may increase further, because

   a. she is demonstrating marked anxiety.
   b. adolescents are usually unprepared for labor.
   c. adolescents have difficulty with authority figures.
   d. her labor will be prolonged.

2. For which of the following patients would administration of analgesia seem most appropriate?

   a. 3 cm, with contractions every 4 to 5 minutes, lasting 30 seconds, and of mild intensity.
   b. 5 cm, with contractions every 3 minutes, lasting 50 seconds, and of moderate to strong intensity; FHR 140 with good variability; patient relaxing well and breathing with contractions.
   c. 7 cm, with contractions every 3 minutes, lasting 50 seconds, and of moderate to strong intensity; FHR 140 with minimal variability and occasional late deceleration.
   d. 7 cm, with contractions every 3 minutes, lasting 50 seconds, and of moderate to strong intensity; FHR 140 with good variability; patient tense and unable to relax between contractions.

3. The physician orders 75 mg of meperidine hydrochloride delivered intramuscularly. You have on hand 100 mg in 2 ml. How much will you administer?

   a. 0.5 mL
   b. 1.0 mL
   c. 1.5 mL
   d. 1.75 mL

4. After administering meperidine hydrochloride to a laboring patient, you should

   a. assess maternal vital signs and the FHR frequently.
   b. assess cervical dilatation every 30 minutes.
   c. turn off the light, close the door, and allow the patient to sleep for a while.
   d. tell the patient that you will not be able to give her anything else because the baby may become addicted.

5. Which of the following observations would indicate a beneficial effect of the meperidine hydrochloride?

   a. The patient dozes between contractions and is able to maintain breathing patterns during contractions. The FHR remains at 140.
   b. Uterine contractions change from every 2½ minutes, lasting 50 seconds, to every 4 minutes, lasting 35 seconds
   c. The FHR baseline is 120 with no deceleration.
   d. The cervical dilatation changes from 7 cm to complete in 30 minutes.

6. Which of the following observations would indicate a side effect of spinal anesthesia?

   a. Numbness of lower trunk and extremities
   b. Diuresis occurring on the second postpartal day
   c. Headache occurring on the first postpartal day
   d. Hypertension in the obstetric recovery room

7. An expected beneficial effect of a paracervical block is

   a. numbness of the lower trunk and extremities
   b. fetal bradycardia
   c. elimination of the bearing-down reflex in the second stage
   d. an anesthetic effect in the cervix and the upper two-thirds of the vagina

8. If the patient exhibited hypotension following a caudal block, you would

   a. do nothing. Hypotension is an expected side effect and requires no treatment.
   b. turn her from the supine to the prone position and administer oxygen.
   c. discontinue intravenous fluids to reduce the chance of fluid overload.
   d. turn her from the supine to the lateral position, administer oxygen, and increase the rate of intravenous fluids.

9. A pudendal block

   a. anesthetizes the lower two-thirds of the vagina and perineum.
   b. anesthetizes the cervix and the upper two-thirds of the vagina.
   c. is frequently associated with fetal bradycardia.
   d. may be given as a continuous block.

10. Neonatal respiratory depression immediately after delivery would most likely be associated with which of the following?

   a. 25 mg of meperidine hydrochloride administered intravenously 3 hours before delivery
   b. 75 mg of meperidine hydrochloride administered intramuscularly 1 hour before delivery
   c. A local anesthetic block
   d. A pudendal block

Answers

1. a   6. c
2. d   7. d
3. c   8. d
4. a   9. a
5. a   10. b

SELECTED BIBLIOGRAPHY

Caritis, S.N., et al. November 1980. Fetal acid-base state following spinal or epidural anesthesia for cesarean section. *Obstet. Gynecol.* 56:610.

Jouppila, P., et al. 1979. Effect of induction of general anesthesia for cesarean section on intervillous blood flow. *Acta Obstet. Gynecol. Scand.* 58:249.

Jouppila, P., et al. December 1979. Epidural analgesia and placental blood flow during labor in pregnancies complicated by hypertension. *Br. J. Obstet. Gynaecol.* 86:969.

Maclaughlin, S.M., and Taubenheim, A.M. January-February 1981. Epidural anesthesia for obstetric patients. *J. Obstet. Gynecol. Neonatal Nurs.* 10:9.

Marx, G.F. October 1979. Analgesia and anesthesia for labor and delivery. *AANA J.* 47:537.

Read, J.A., and Miller, F.C. February 1979. The bupivocaine paracervical block in labor and its effect on quantitative uterine activity. *Obstet. Gyencol.* 53:166.

CHAPTER 11 COMPLICATIONS OF THE INTRAPARTAL PERIOD

INTRODUCTION

As her pregnancy advances, each woman wonders about the course of her labor and delivery. A relatively smooth labor and delivery with a healthy baby is, of course, the desired outcome and is the result in the majority of cases. However, in some instances problems develop that complicate the process of birth and jeopardize the well-being of mother or baby or both. Early, accurate assessment of potential problems and appropriate therapeutic interventions are the key to achieving the best outcome possible.

This chapter focuses on the complications that may arise during labor and delivery. Attention is given to the etiology and clinical picture in order to assist the nurse in patient assessment. Implications for both mother and fetus are also presented when appropriate. Anticipated interventions are then presented. Using this knowledge, the nurse will be able to evaluate the effectiveness of the patient's care.

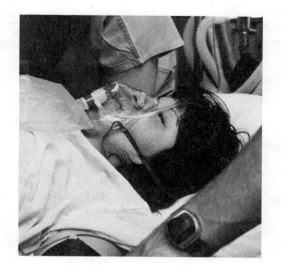

PART I
GENERAL PRINCIPLES AND CONCEPTS

1. Compare the dysfunctional labor patterns in the chart on page 192.

192

PATTERN	CAUSE	MONITOR TRACING	IMPLICATIONS	INTERVENTIONS	COMPLICATIONS
Hypertonic			Maternal		
			Fetal		
Hypotonic			Maternal		
			Fetal		
Prolonged			Maternal		
			Fetal		
Precipitous			Maternal		
			Fetal		

Preterm Labor

2. Define *preterm labor*.

3. List three maternal causative factors that may be associated with preterm labor.
   a.

   b.

   c.

4. List three fetal causative factors that may be associated with preterm labor.
   a.

   b.

   c.

5. Explain the implications of preterm labor for the fetus.

6. List four conditions that would preclude interruption of preterm labor.*
   a.

   b.

*These questions are addressed at the end of Part I.

c.

d.

7. At this time, ritodrine is approved by the Federal Drug Administration for use in the treatment of preterm labor. Terbutaline sulfate is also in use as part of a treatment regimen for this condition. In the following chart the last column has been provided to encourage you to analyze any additional medication that is commonly used in your region.

CHARACTERISTIC	RITODRINE (Yutopar)	TERBUTALINE SULFATE (Brethine)	OTHER
a. Mechanism of action			
b. Administration (route and dosage)			
c. Maternal side effects*			
d. Fetal side effects			

*These questions are addressed at the end of Part I.

CHARACTERISTIC	RITODRINE (Yutopar)	TERBUTALINE SULFATE (Brethine)	OTHER
e. Nursing interventions*			

8. Why may the obstetrician order electrocardiogram and serum potassium for a patient receiving ritodrine intravenously?

9. Patients who are receiving a maintenance dose of ritodrine may also be given betamethasone intramuscularly. Explain the desired effect of betamethasone administration.

Complications Involving the Fetus

10. Complete the following chart, which addresses four types of fetal malposition/malpresentations:

FETAL MALPOSITION/ MALPRESEN- TATION	SIGNS AND SYMPTOMS	MATERNAL IMPLICATIONS	FETAL/ NEONATAL IMPLICATIONS	INTERVENTIONS
Occiput posterior position				
Face presentation				

*These questions are addressed at the end of Part I.

FETAL MALPOSITION/ MALPRESEN-TATION	SIGNS AND SYMPTOMS	MATERNAL IMPLICATIONS	FETAL/ NEONATAL IMPLICATIONS	INTERVENTIONS
Brow presentation				
Transverse lie				

CPD (cephalopelvic disproportion) may accompany a malpresentation or malposition of the fetus, a large fetus, or abnormalities in the maternal pelvis.

11. List two clinical manifestations during labor that may indicate CPD.

    a.

    b.

12. How can a woman with possible CPD be evaluated?

13. Explain the rationale for allowing a "trial of labor" for a woman with borderline pelvic measurements.

14. Meleah Stone, gravida III, para II, is admitted with contractions every 2 minutes, lasting 60 seconds and of strong intensity. Her membranes ruptured spontaneously 2 hours ago, and Meleah reports that the fluid has been "greenish." She is breathing well with contractions and denies any discomfort. When assessing FHR, you located it above the umbilicus, at 140 beats per minute and regular. What would you suspect?*

15. Explain the possible reasons for the presence of greenish amniotic fluid. What special measures will need to be taken for the newborn immediately after delivery due to the presence of the green-stained fluid?*

16. Define the following types of breech presentations:

    a. Frank breech

    b. Complete breech

    c. Footling breech

17. What is the rationale for using forceps during a breech delivery?

18. What type of forceps may be used during a breech delivery?*

*These questions are addressed at the end of Part I.

Multiple Pregnancy and Twins

19. Lisa Rote is in her second pregnancy. List two signs and symptoms that may indicate the presence of twins.

    a.

    b.

20. Identify three implications for Lisa of the multiple pregnancy.

    a.

    b.

    c.

21. Discuss the implications of the multiple pregnancy for the fetuses during labor and delivery.*

22. The major maternal complication that may occur following delivery of twins is _____. This occurs because _____.

Fetal Distress

23. List three signs and symptoms that would indicate fetal distress.*

    a.

---

*These questions are addressed at the end of Part I.

b. Describe the immediate nursing acts indicated in this situation. Include the rationale.

c.

24. Describe the general nursing measures that can be taken in case of fetal distress. Include your rationale.

    a.

    b.

    c.

    d.

25. Ann Kelley has been in active labor for 4 hours. She states that her membranes have just ruptured. As you prepare to do a vaginal examination, you notice the umbilical cord protruding from her vagina.

    a. What does this signify?

b. Describe the immediate nursing actions indicated in this situation. Include the rationale.

Placental Problems

26. Define *abruptio placentae*.

27. Describe the clinical manifestations of the following:

a. Overt (marginal) placental abruption

b. Covert (central) placental abruption

    c. Placental prolapse (complete separation)

28. Discuss the implications of abruptio placentae.

    a. For the mother

    b. For the fetus/neonate

29. List five nursing measures for the patient with abruptio placentae. Include your rationale.

    a.

    b.

c.

d.

e.

30. Define *placenta previa*.

31. List the three types of placenta previa.

    a.

    b.

    c.

32. Describe the clinical manifestations of placenta previa.

33. List two maternal implications of placenta previa.

    a.

    b.

34. List two fetal/neonatal implications of placenta previa.

    a.

    b.

35. Dortha Haney, gravida III, para I, is admitted to the labor deck with moderate vaginal bleeding. She is at 39 weeks' gestation. She states that she is not having contractions but that she has had episodes of vaginal bleeding since the 20th week. An ultrasound reading demonstrated a marginal placenta previa. The FHR is 140. You know that a vaginal examination is usually done as patients are admitted to assess cervical dilatation. Will you do a vaginal examination on Dortha? Give the rationale for your answer.

36. Identify two methods that may be used to diagnose placenta previa.

    a.

    b.

37. Describe appropriate medical and nursing interventions for the patient with placenta previa.

38. Disseminated intravascular coagulation (DIC) is a potential complication of abruptio placentae and placenta previa. Why may this develop?

Hydramnios

39. Hydramnios occurs when there is more than _____ mL of amniotic fluid in the uterus.

40. Polly Brooks is diagnosed as having hydramnios. List three implications of this diagnosis for her prenatal course.

    a.

    b.

    c.

41. Identify three implications of hydramnios for the fetus.*

    a.

    b.

    c.

42. Polly's baby is born with esophageal atresia. Why is this more frequently seen in cases of hydramnios?

Oligohydramnios

43. Define *oligohydramnios*.

44. The major maternal complication of oligohydramnios is _____.*

44. Explain why oligohydramnios may be present when the fetus has a malformation or malfunction of the genitourinary system.

Forceps Delivery

46. List three indications for the use of forceps to assist in vaginal delivery.

   a.

   b.

   c.

*These questions are addressed at the end of Part I.

47. Identify the criteria that should be met in order to safely use forceps.

48. Define the following:

    a. Low forceps delivery

    b. Midforceps delivery

49. Identify complications (maternal and fetal) that may be associated with forceps delivery.

50. Identify the nursing interventions that are necessary during a low forceps (outlet) delivery.*

Selected Answers

This section addresses the asterisked questions found in this chapter.

6. Preterm labor would not be interrupted in the presence of

    a. active labor and cervical dilatation of 4 cm or more.

    b. ruptured amniotic membranes, with maternal fever.

    c. such fetal complications as isoimmunization.

    d. such maternal complications as severe preeclampsia-eclampsia.

7. c. The maternal side effects of ritodrine include tachycardia, hypotension, increased blood glucose and insulin, increased free fatty acids, decreased serum potassium, palpitations, tremor, nausea, vomiting, headache, erythema, nervousness, chest pain, dyspnea, cardiac arrhythmias, and pulmonary edema.

    The maternal side effects of terbutaline include tachycardia, nervousness, tremors, headache, nausea, vomiting, palpitations, drowsiness, hypotension, and pulmonary edema.

    e. Nursing interventions for a woman on intravenous ritodrine should unclude the following:

        encourage the woman to lie on her left side (to decrease the incidence of hypotension from pressure of the gravid uterus on the vena cava).

        use a fetal monitor for continuous tracing.

        watch for signs of a toxic dosage level in the woman and fetus.

        record intake and output and intravenous fluid intake.

        assess the maternal pulse and the FHR every 10 minutes until the effective dosage level is reached. Then assess them every 2 hours (at a minimum).

        notify the physician if the maternal pulse is greater than 120 beats per minute and/or the FHR is greater than 180 beats per minute.

        assess uterine contractions.

        assess blood pressure hourly while intravenous infusion is taking place.

        assess the laboratory reports of serum electrolytes.

        assess the woman's respiratory status.

        assess the woman for cardiac arrhythmias.

        do not use an intravenous ritodrine solution if it is discolored or contains a precipitate.

        if symptoms of an overdose are severe with intravenous ritodrine infusion, the infusion must be discontinued. A beta blocking agent may be given as an antidote.

*These questions are addressed at the end of Part I.

The above interventions are specifically directed toward the ritodrine therapy. Many additional nursing interventions could be addressed for a patient in preterm labor.

The nursing interventions for a patient on intravenous terbutaline sulfate are very similar to those listed for intravenous ritodrine.

14. You should expect a breech presentation.
15. When the fetus is in a breech presentation, there may be a release of meconium due to the pressures occurring during contractions. In this instance the release of meconium would most likely be viewed as physiologic. However, the possibility of fetal distress must be considered.

When there is evidence of meconium staining of the amniotic fluid during labor, the delivery room team needs to be prepared to remove secretions from the newborn's naso-oropharynx immediately after birth. A DeLee trap is frequently used to remove these secretions. In the case of a breech presentation, the newborn will be suctioned as soon as the head is delivered. In vertex presentations, the naso-oropharynx is suctioned as soon as the head appears, and before the first breath is taken, so the secretions are not drawn into the lungs with the first breath. If the newborn continues to demonstrate distress, the vocal cords will be visualized with a laryngoscope. If meconium is seen, suctioning will be done. Aspiration of meconium can result in meconium-aspiration pneumonia in the early neonatal period.

18. Piper forceps are commonly used during a breech delivery.
21. Implications for the fetuses may include

    a. inadequate nourishment of one fetus during gestation.
    b. premature labor, with associated problems of respiratory distress syndrome.
    c. difficulty in evaluating whether the second fetus can be delivered vaginally if the first fetus is delivered breech.
    d. interlocked fetuses.
    e. slow or interrupted labor because of overstretching of the uterus.

23. Fetal distress would be indicated by any of the following:

    a. severe late or variable decelerations
    b. severe bradycardia
    c. meconium staining in a vertex presentation
    d. cessation of movement
    e. hyperactive fetal movement
    f. loss of variability

41. Polyhydramnios may be associated with

    a. an increased incidence of fetal malformations
    b. premature labor
    c. fetal malpresentation
    d. prolapse of the cord when the membranes rupture

44. The major maternal complication of oligohydramnios is dysfunctional labor.
50. The nursing interventions that are necessary during a low forceps delivery include the following:

    a. Explain the procedure to the woman and her support person.
    b. Encourage the woman to maintain her breathing pattern during application of the forceps. (Panting may help to relieve the "need to push" sensation that she will feel as the forceps are applied.)
    c. Monitor the FHR continuously.
    d. Monitor contractions. Inform the physician when a contraction begins and ends, because he or she will exert downward pressure on the forceps during a contraction.
    e. Provide support to the woman throughout the process.
    f. Ensure that adequate resuscitation equipment is available and in working order before the delivery.
    g. After delivery, assess the newborn for the Apgar score; facial bruising, swelling, abrasions, and/or paralysis; signs of cerebral trauma; and movement of arms (to detect paralysis).

PART II
SELF-ASSESSMENT GUIDE

The following multiple-choice questions will help you assess your knowledge of the content of this chapter. Select the best answer for each of the questions and then refer to the end of Part II to check your answers.

1. Signs and symptoms of the patient with hyperactive labor would include all of the following *except*

   a. contractions every 2 minutes, lasting 90 seconds.
   b. rapid progressive cervical dilatation.
   c. a prolonged active phase.
   d. discomfort that seems out of proportion to the uterine contractions.

2. A primigravida is admitted at term in early labor. You note on her prenatal record that her pelvic measurements are diagonal conjugate 10 cm, biischial diameter 7 cm. Based on this information, you would expect her labor to be

   a. within the normal length of time for primigravidas.
   b. prolonged, with slow fetal descent.
   c. prolonged, with failure of the fetal head to engage.
   d. "normal" through the first stage and prolonged pushing in the second stage.

3. Vicky Brookens is at 34 weeks' gestation and is on intravenous ritodrine. She complains of nervousness. Her blood pressure has changed from 120/80 to 100/70. Her pulse rate is 154. Based on your knowledge of ritodrine, you will

   a. assess for bleeding because of the signs of impending shock.
   b. call the physician to report the decreased blood pressure and increased pulse.
   c. continue to follow your labor and delivery protocol, because all signs and symptoms are normal for ritodrine therapy.
   d. encourage Vicky to relax, because her nervousness is affecting her vital signs.

4. In which of the following situations would it be possible to perform a low (outlet) forceps delivery?

   a. When the head is ballottable
   b. When the head reaches the perineal floor
   c. When the occiput is at the ischial spines
   d. When the biparietal diameter of the head reaches the pelvic inlet

5. The severe abdominal pain that may be associated with abruptio placentae is due to

   a. retroplacental collection of blood.
   b. precipitous labor.
   c. bleeding into the peritoneal cavity.
   d. marginal separation of the placenta.

6. A patient with partial placenta previa delivers following a 3-hour labor. The complication she is *most* likely to develop in the early postpartal period is

   a. hemorrhage.
   b. infection.
   c. hypofibrinogenemia.
   d. couvelaire uterus.

7. A 20-year-old primigravida is admitted at term. She has a moderate amount of dark vaginal bleeding. Uterine contractions are every 3 minutes lasting 40 seconds. The FHR is 140. Based on this information, you would know that

   a. you should suspect abruptio placentae.
   b. she is experiencing "normal" labor.
   c. she is near the end of the first stage.
   d. you should obtain an order for an analgesic.

8. A patient who has a breech presentation might have which of the following?

   a. A greater amount of bloody show during labor
   b. Slower labor progress than the norm
   c. More intense labor contractions
   d. A precipitous labor

9. While performing a vaginal examination, you note a glistening white cord protruding from the vagina. Your *first* nursing action would be to

   a. return to the nurse's station to place an emergency call to the physician.
   b. start administering oxygen by mask at 4 L per minute and assess the mother's vital signs.
   c. place a clean towel over the cord and wet it with a sterile normal saline solution.
   d. apply manual pressure to the presenting part and have the mother assume a knee-chest position.

10. You know that your initial nursing action for the situation in question 9 is effective when you find that

   a. the FHR is maintained at 140.
   b. there is no vaginal bleeding.
   c. the mother does not develop an infection.
   d. the mother's vital signs stay within a normal range.

Answers

1. c	6. a
2. c	7. a
3. b	8. b
4. b	9. d
5. a	10. a

SELECTED BIBLIOGRAPHY

Ballas, S., et al. July 1979. Midtrimester placenta previa: normal or pathologic finding. *Obstet. Gynecol.* 54:6.

Bills, B.J. July-August 1980. Nursing considerations: administering labor-suppressing medications. *MCN.* 5:252.

Cederquist, L.L., et al. April 1980. Effect of glucocorticoids on fetal immunoglobulin production after premature rupture of membranes, *Obstet. Gynecol.* 55:444.

Crout, T.K. April 1980. Caring for the mother of a stillborn baby. *Nurs. 80.* 10:70.

Douvas, S.G., and Morrison, J.C. December 1982. A guide to OB emergencies. *Contemp. OB/GYN.* 20:95.

Friedman, E.A. February 1983. Whither midforceps? Its place in OB today. *Contemp. OB/GYN.* 21:85.

Gimovsky, M.L., and Petrie, R.H. April 1983. Strategy for choosing the best delivery route for the breech baby. *Contemp. OB/GYN.* 21:201.

Ingemarsson, E., et al. March 1980. Influence of occiput posterior position on the fetal heart rate pattern. *Obstet. Gynecol.* 55:301.

Jennings, B. May-June 1979. Emergency delivery: how to attend to one safely. *MCN.* 4:148.

Merkatz, I.R. July 1980. Ritodrine hydrochloride: a betamimetic agent for use in pre-term labor. I. Pharmacology, clinical history, administration, side effects and safety. *Obstet. Gynecol.* 56:1.

Modanlou, H.D., et al. April 1980. Macrosomia: maternal, fetal, and neonatal implications. *Obstet. Gynecol.* 55:420.

Notelovitz, M., et al. February 1979. Painless abruptio placentae. *Obstet. Gynecol.* 53:270.

Read, J.A. November 1980. Urinary bladder distention: effect on labor and uterine activity. *Obstet. Gynecol.* 56:565.

Shearer, E.C. Spring 1982. Education for vaginal birth after Cesarean Birth. *Birth*. 9:31.

Spaulding, L.B., and Gallup, D.G. October 1979. Current concepts of management of rupture of the gravid uterus. *Obstet. Gynecol*. 54:437.

Varner, M.W. September 1980. X-ray pelvimetry in clinical obstetrics. *Obstet. Gynecol*. 56:296.

Vice, L.J. September-October 1979. Touching the high-risk obstetrical patient. *J. Obstet. Gynecol. Neonatal Nurs*. 8:294.

Wexler, P., and Gottesfeld, K.R. August 1979. Early diagnosis of placenta previa. *Obstet. Gynecol*. 54:231.

CHAPTER 12 *NURSING ASSESSMENT AND CARE OF THE POSTPARTAL FAMILY*

INTRODUCTION

The puerperium is a time of major physiologic and psychologic adaptations as the body completes its adjustment following delivery. This chapter begins with questions on theoretical data about common physiologic and psychologic changes. The remainder of the chapter emphasizes clinical application of the nursing process in providing care for the postpartal family.

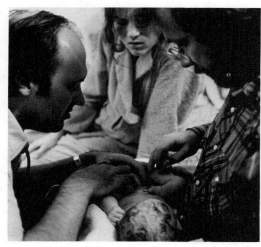

PART I
GENERAL PRINCIPLES AND CONCEPTS

Physical Adaptations

1. Complete the following chart:

PHYSIOLOGIC FEATURE	EXPECTED CHANGES	PHYSIOLOGIC RATIONALE
Uterus	Size	
	Muscle tone	
	Placental site	

PHYSIOLOGIC FEATURE	EXPECTED CHANGES	PHYSIOLOGIC RATIONALE
Uterus	Lochia	
	Lochia Odor	
	Amount	
Cervix		
Vagina		
Perineum		
Abdomen		
Urinary tract	Kidneys	
	Ureters	

PHYSIOLOGIC FEATURE	EXPECTED CHANGES	PHYSIOLOGIC RATIONALE
Urinary tract	Bladder	
	Urinary output	
Gastrointestinal tract		
Breasts		
Vital signs		
Blood values		
Weight changes		

2. Explain the physiologic mechanisms and time of onset involved in the following:
   a. Postpartal chills

b. Postpartal diaphoresis

c. Afterpains

Clinical Application

3. Identify nine areas that should be examined during the initial postpartal physical assessment and then at least daily until the client is discharged. (Do not include psychologic assessment or information needs.)*

a.

b.

c.

d.

e.

f.

g.

h.

i.

*These questions are addressed at the end of Part I.

4. Describe three observations you should make in assessing the breasts of a postpartal client. Include your rationale for each.

   a.

   b.

   c.

5. Describe the physiology of breast engorgement.

6. On her third postpartal day, Erika Timm, who is not breast-feeding, complains of feelings of fullness and discomfort in her breasts. In addition to the administration of medication to suppress lactation, list at least four nursing measures that may be taken to help ease her discomfort.

   a.

   b.

   c.

   d.

7. List at least five points to be included in a teaching plan to help Erika successfully bottle-feed her infant.

   a.

   b.

   c.

d.

e.

8. Allison Reed, a breast-feeding mother, also complains of engorgement. List five measures that may be taken to ease her discomfort.

   a.

   b.

   c.

   d.

   e.

9. Pamela is attempting to breast-feed her first infant and asks for your assistance. She has numerous questions about all aspects of breast-feeding. What information would you give her about each of the following?

   a. Let-down reflex

   b. Nipple care

   c. Breast support

    d. Frequency of feeding

    e. Length of time per breast

    f. Positions for feeding

    g. Methods for getting the baby to begin nursing

    h. Breaking suction before removing the infant from the breast

    i. Measures for relieving sore nipples

    j. Use of supplementary feedings

k. Manual expression of breast milk

l. Maternal nutrition while breast-feeding

m. Use of medications while breast-feeding

n. Environmental influences

o. Personal support system

p. Available community resources

10. What observations of Pamela and her infant during feeding would indicate that your teaching has been effective?

11. During your discussion with her, Pamela mentions that her girlfriend told her that eating any chocolate was absolutely forbidden as long as she was breast-feeding. How might you respond to this?

12. On her third postpartal day, Pamela expresses concern: "My breast milk used to be so creamy and yellow. Now it looks so watery, almost like skim milk. Do you think my diet is lacking?" How might you respond to this?

As part of your postpartum assessment, you palpate your client's abdomen.

13. Define *diastasis rectus abdominis*. How does it occur, and how is it measured?

14. Why is it necessary to assess the fundus following delivery?

   a. What is the significance of a well-contracted uterus?

   b. Why is the client asked to empty her bladder before you assess her fundus?

   c. Describe the correct procedure for evaluating descent of the fundus.

   d. How is fundal height recorded (according to your agency's policy)?

15. It is the second postpartal day for Megan Davenport, a 21-year-old primipara. Yesterday her fundus was one finger breadth below the umbilicus. Where would you expect it to be today? _____

16. What characteristics should be noted in assessing Megan's lochia?

17. How do you record your findings about the lochia (according to your agency's policy)?

18. When getting up to go to the bathroom after awakening on her second postpartal day, Megan becomes alarmed when she notices a sudden increase in her lochia. You check her fundus and it is firm. How might you explain this ocurrence?

19. In preparation for assessing Megan's perineum, you would have her assume the _____ position.

20. List and explain the significance of the components of the REEDA scale in evaluating the condition of the episiotomy.

COMPONENT	SIGNIFICANCE
R_____	
E_____	
E_____	
D_____	
A_____	

21. What observations about the condition of any hemorrhoids should be made during the assessment of the perineum?

22. What information regarding the client's urinary elimination should be elicited during your physical assessment?

23. You find your client's uterus at one finger breadth above the umbilicus and displaced to the right side.

    a. What would you suspect?

    b. What further assessments should you make?

    c. What nursing actions will you take?

    d. What observations would you make to evaluate the effectiveness of your nursing actions?

24. You are assisting Edna Lewis to the bathroom for the first time following delivery.

    a. What nursing assessments should you make before Edna gets up?

    b. What teaching regarding perineal hygiene should you initiate at this time?

25. Edna has difficulty voiding.

    a. Explain why voiding may be difficult following delivery.

    b. List nursing measures you might use to assist Edna in voiding.

    c. How would you evaluate the effectiveness of your nursing actions?

26. What information about the client's intestinal elimination should you elicit during your physical examination?

27. Discuss the teaching implications of your findings on intestinal elimination.

28. Why is it important to include an evaluation of a client's lower extremities as part of your postpartal assessment?

29. How is Homan's sign elicited?

30. What assessments are important in evaluating your client's nutritional status?

31. One of your clients is a 28-year-old lactating mother of average weight.

    a. What are her nutritional needs?

    b. Prepare a daily menu for her if she is of:

        ANGLO DESCENT   **HISPANIC DESCENT**†

†You may substitute an ethnic background common to your locale.

32. Another client is a 16-year-old lactating mother.

   a. What nutritional teaching is indicated for her?

   b. If she asks you for advice on losing weight while she is nursing, how will you respond?

33. Listed below are the major sources of discomfort for the postpartal client. For each discomfort, identify comfort measures that may be instituted and the rationale for each.

DISCOMFORT	COMFORT MEASURES	RATIONALE
Episiotomy		
Hemorrhoids		
Afterpains		

34. How will a cesarean delivery affect the postpartal nursing assessment and care of a client?

35. During the postpartal period, you may be asked to administer several of the drugs listed in the following chart. For each drug, state the action/use, dose, side effects/untoward effects, and nursing considerations. Space has also been provided for you to add drugs commonly used in your agency.

DRUG[†]	ACTION/USE	DOSE	EXCRE- TION IN BREAST MILK	SIDE EFFECTS/ UNTOWARD EFFECTS	NURSING CONSIDERATIONS
Methergine					
Tace					
Parlodel					
Dialose					
Surfak					
Annusol HC suppository					
Ferrous sulfate					
Empirin #3					
Percodan					
RhoGAM					
Rubella vaccine					

[†]This list is a sample. You are encouraged to substitute any drugs that are commonly used on your unit.

36. Identify factors that influence a new mother's psychologic adjustment to her delivery and newborn.

37. Reva Rubin has described two major stages of adjustment during the early postpartal period: the taking-in phase and the taking-hold phase. Briefly discuss each, with emphasis on the maternal behaviors that are exhibited and their significance for nursing care.

    a. Taking-in phase

    b. Taking-hold phase

38. Briefly describe the "postpartum blues" and the nursing interventions that are indicated for clients experiencing them.

39. Freda and Earl Marshall express concern about the possible reaction of their 3-year-old son, Roy, to the birth of their daughter. Briefly describe some actions they might take to help Roy more easily adjust to the arrival of his sister.

40. Freda asks you about postpartal exercises. Develop an appropriate exercise plan and specify on which postpartal day each exercise may begin.

41. Freda asks when she and her husband can resume sexual activity. How would you respond?

42. Freda is breast-feeding her baby and tells you that her friend told her that breast-feeding is a natural, effective method of birth control. How would you respond?

43. You are discussing contraception with a group of postpartal mothers. Complete the following chart:

CONTRACEPTIVE METHOD	MECHANISM OF ACTION	SIDE EFFECTS/ UNTOWARD EFFECTS	RELIABILITY	PATIENT TEACHING
Oral contraceptives				
Intrauterine device				
Diaphragm				
Cervical cap				
Foams, jellies, vaginal suppositories, and condoms				
Coitus interruptus				

CONTRACEPTIVE METHOD	MECHANISM OF ACTION	SIDE EFFECTS/ UNTOWARD EFFECTS	RELIABILITY	PATIENT TEACHING
Postcoital douche				
Fertility awareness methods				

44. Rooming-in is expanding in popularity.

   a. Define *rooming-in*.

   b. Explain the advantages for the mother who is rooming-in.

   c. Explain the disadvantages for the mother.

   d. Explain the nursing responsibilities in caring for the mother and newborn during the rooming-in experience.

232

45. In many postpartal units the focus of care and attention is the mother and her newborn. Describe how you would incorporate the father or support person into your focus of care.*

46. In addition to her name, age, and social history, what information would you consider essential to have as part of your data base in planning care for a postpartal client?*

47. Carla Roberts, age 29, gravida III para II, delivered an 8 lb 7 oz boy at 3:15 AM. Her labor lasted 18 hours, and the baby was delivered by low forceps. She received no medication during labor but did have a pudendal block for delivery. She had a midline episiotomy and a third-degree extension. She also has two large hemorrhoids. The baby had an Apgar score of 7 at 1 minute and 9 at 5 minutes. He is apparently healthy, although he has a large bruise on each temple from the forceps and pronounced molding of his head. The labor and delivery nurse reported that Harry Roberts, Carla's husband, was present at the birth and expressed great pleasure at the birth of his third son. Carla was openly disappointed that the newborn was not the girl she had so greatly desired.

It is now 8 AM. Carla has just finished breakfast, and you are assigned as her nurse today. Carla has voided twice since delivery: 700 mL and 550 mL. Her fundus has remained firm and is at the umbilicus. Her lochia is rubra and moderate. Her vital signs are normal, and she is a breast-feeding mother. Her orders include: a shower; a sitz bath TID; Dermaplast spray prn.; up ad lib.; Tylenol # 3 q4h. prn.; a regular diet; encourage fluids; a straight catheter × 1 prn for marked distention; and Surfak 1 capsule BID.

a. What do you consider the two highest priorities in planning Carla's physical care?*

*These questions are addressed at the end of Part I.

b. Develop a plan of care for the morning based on your assessment of Carla's condition. Include the appropriate rationale.
    Patient care goals:

PROBLEM/NEED	NURSING ACTION	RATIONALE

Nursing care evaluation:

c. You know that disappointment over the sex of an infant may produce problems in maternal-infant bonding. Identify two ways that you can assess Carla for potential bonding problems.*

*These questions are addressed at the end of Part I.

    d. In observing Carla with her new son, what behaviors might she exhibit that would indicate healthy maternal-infant bonding?

    e. What behaviors might Carla exhibit that would suggest possible failure to bond well?

48. Vicky and Larry Darnell are preparing to take their first child, Lori, home today. Vicky is planning to bottle-feed Lori. Vicky had an uncomplicated labor and delivery but has a small midline episiotomy that has caused some discomfort. You are assigned to Mrs. Darnell today and are responsible for discharge teaching. Describe what information you will include in your discharge teaching for the following areas:

    a. Care of the episiotomy

    b. Sitz baths

    c. Rest

    d. Activity and exercises

    e. Resumption of sexual activity and birth control methods

f. Symptoms that should be reported

g. Support systems

h. Diapering the baby

i. Bathing the baby

j. Cord care

k. Formula preparation

l. Safety (crib, car seat)

m. Followup medical care for both mother and infant

n. Community resources

49. Naomi Carlson has delivered her first child in the birthing room and has spent the 24 hours since delivery in the postpartal unit. She is preparing to go home with her newborn today.

   a. Describe how you will explain the reasons for and the importance of returning to the hospital for a phenylketonuria test.

   b. You will be accompanying the registered nurse on a home visit to Naomi's home tomorrow. List the assessments you will need to make on your home visit.*

MOTHER	NEWBORN	EDUCATIONAL NEEDS

Selected Answers

This section addresses the asterisked questions found in this chapter.

3. The following essential areas need to be included in your daily physical assessment of the postpartal client.

   a. vital signs
   b. breasts, including nipples
   c. fundus and abdomen
   d. lochia
   e. perineum (including the anus)
   f. elimination
   g. lower extremities
   h. nutritional status
   i. activity level

   If you listed most of these, you are well on your way to providing good nursing care for your clients. If you missed three or more, you need to refer back to the postpartum section in your textbook. Other areas that may be considered are the discomfort level and sleep patterns.

45. The father can be included more readily by

   a. encouraging him to visit whenever possible during the day or evening and to participate in infant care.
   b. encouraging him to come in for infant feeding.
   c. including him in parenting classes in the postpartal unit.

*These questions are addressed at the end of Part I.

d. being supportive of his efforts.

e. providing time for him to ask any questions that he might have.

f. including him in all teaching.

These are just a few possibilities. You may have thought of others.

46. You should include information about her obstetric history, including the following:

a. number of pregnancies, births, and abortions

b. significant prenatal problems and conditions

c. delivery date and time

d. medications given (anesthesia and analgesics)

e. course of labor and delivery (for example, time of rupture of membranes; use of forceps, episiotomy, prolonged second stage)

f. sex, Apgar score, and present condition of the infant, along with pertinent recovery room data

g. available support systems (In many agencies the mother's marital status has little relevance. The focus is on the support she has available to her.)

h. any existing problems or complaints (including allergies to food and drugs)

i. method of feeding the infant

j. teaching needs

If you included most of this information, you are on the right track. If you included the physical aspects but neglected the support and teaching areas, you may find it helpful to review material related to psychologic adjustments and teaching needs during the early postpartal period.

47. a. High on your list of priorities in planning Carla's physical care you should include a need for rest and a need for comfort. With an 18-hour labor, you know that she has been up all night and most of the preceding day. Her third-degree extension and hemorrhoids make comfort important, and meeting this need will enable her to rest more easily.

Because this is probably her first shower, safety is a fairly high priority, as it is with most patients following delivery.

If you listed bladder or intestinal elimination as a high priority, you may wish to review your textbook.

It is always pertinent to assess a postpartal patient for hemorrhage, but since her fundus has remained firm, it would not be your highest priority.

c. You can assess Carla's attitude toward her child by unobtrusively observing her with her infant and by discussing the subject with her in an open, nonjudgmental way.

Although her history suggests a possible bonding problem, it is not appropriate to jump to conclusions without further data. Frequently parents will express initial disappointment about a child's sex or behavior and then bond beautifully later.

49. b. The postpartal home visit should include assessment of the following:

MOTHER	NEWBORN	EDUCATIONAL NEEDS
Vital signs	Vital signs	Self-care
Breasts	Skin color and rashes	Baby care
Fundus	Umbilical cord	
Lochia	Feedings	
Episiotomy	Voiding and stooling pattern	
Bladder	Sleep pattern	
Bowels	Alertness	
Rest and nutrition		
Mother-infant interaction		
Support systems		

Congratulations if you included all (or most) of these items. If you had trouble with this question, you need to refer to the postpartal assessment guide in your textbook.

PART II
SELF-ASSESSMENT GUIDE

The following multiple-choice questions will help you assess your knowledge of the content of this chapter. Select the best answer for each of the questions then refer to the end of Part II to check your answers.

Questions 1-6 pertain to the following situation. Joyce Palmer, a 24-year-old gravida I para I, delivered Bryan, an 8-lb full-term infant. She is nursing her infant. She had a midline episiotomy. It is her second postpartal day. As part of your daily postpartal care, you assess each of the following systems for signs that they are functioning normally.

1. The fundus should be

    a. soft and at the level of the symphysis pubis.
    b. firm and midway between the umbilicus and symphysis pubis.
    c. soft and at the level of the umbilicus.
    d. firm and two finger breadths below the umbilicus.

2. The lochia should have a

    a. characteristic foul odor and blood mixed with a small amount of mucus.
    b. characteristic foul odor and be dark brown with occasional red bleeding.
    c. fleshy odor and be clear-colored and moderate in amount.
    d. fleshy odor with blood and a small amount of mucus mixed in.

3. The perineum should be

    a. edematous, painful to pressure, and displaying a clear discharge.
    b. edematous, painful to pressure, and perhaps displaying hemorrhoids.
    c. intensely painful in the episiotomy area and displaying clear drainage.
    d. displaying clear drainage and perhaps hemorrhoids.

4. The breasts should be

    a. full and secreting colostrum.
    b. engorged and secreting colostrum.
    c. soft and secreting milk.
    d. engorged and not secreting any fluid.

5. You are instructing Joyce about measures to help relieve her progressive breast discomfort. Which of the following would you suggest to her?

    a. Application of ice packs to the breasts
    b. Application of a firm breast binder to compress the breasts
    c. Application of a warm moist towel and an uplifting support binder or good support brassiere
    d. Decreased fluid intake and application of an uplifting support binder or good support brassiere

6. Which of the following instructions should you give to Joyce about breast care?

    a. Wash your nipples with a mild antiseptic prior to each feeding.
    b. Wash before each feeding with a mild soap.
    c. Wash the nipples once a day with plain water.
    d. Wash nipples daily with warm water and mild soap.

7. Uterine involution ocurs as a result of

    a. a decrease in the number of myometrial cells.
    b. necrosis of the hypertrophic myometrial cells.
    c. autolysis of protein material within the uterine wall.
    d. necrotic degeneration of the placental site.

8. Mrs. Thompson is a gravida II para II. While assessing her fundus 12 hours after delivery, you find that it is enlarged and soft. What would be your first nursing intervention?

    a. Take her vital signs.
    b. Check the consistency of her fundus at 15-minute intervals.
    c. Administer an oxytocic drug.
    d. Massage the uterus firmly with one hand while supporting it with the other hand.

9. Which of the following instructions should be given to a postpartal mother about perineal care?

    a. Cleansing the area should be a sterile procedure.
    b. The area should be cleansed from front to back.
    c. A sterilized perineal pad should be applied to the perineum.
    d. An antiseptic should be used to cleanse the perineum to prevent inflammation.

10. Difficulty in voiding after delivery may be due to which of the following factors?

    a. Decreased sensitivity of the bladder
    b. Lack of food and fluid intake during labor
    c. Relaxation of the abdominal wall
    d. All of the above

11. Mrs. Thomas, a gravida I para I, is planning on bottle-feeding Jennifer. She knows that Jennifer should be allowed to set her own schedule but asks how often that will be. Infants need to have formula approximately how many times a day?

    a. Two to four
    b. Four to six
    c. Six to eight
    d. Eight to ten

12. The taking-in phase of puerperinium occurs during the first 2-3 days after delivery. During this time, the mother is most concerned with

    a. details of her delivery and herself.
    b. discharge plans.
    c. infant care.
    d. postpartal exercises for herself.

Answers

1.	d	7.	c
2.	d	8.	d
3.	b	9.	b
4.	a	10.	d
5.	c	11.	c
6.	c	12.	a

SELECTED BIBLIOGRAPHY

Arafat, I., et al. March-April 1981. Maternal practice and attitudes toward breast feeding. *J. Obstet. Gynecol. Neonatal Nurs.* 10:91.

Beske, J.E. May-June 1982. Important factors in breastfeeding success. *MCN.* 7:174.

Burbach, C.A. September-October 1980. Contraception and adolescent pregnancy. *J. Obstet. Gynecol. Neonatal Nurs.* 9:319.

Carr, K.C., and Walton, V.E. January-February 1982. Early postpartum discharge. *J. Obstet. Gynecol. Neonatal Nurs.* 11:29.

Crowder, D.S. January-February 1981. Maternity nurses' knowledge of factors promoting successful breast feeding: a survey at two hospitals. *J. Obstet. Gynecol. Neonatal Nurs.* 10:28.

Curry, M.A. March-April 1983. Variables related to adaptation to motherhood in "normal" primiparous women. *J. Obstet. Gynecol. Neonatal Nurs.* 12(2):115.

Dickerson, P.S. March-April 1981. Early postpartum separation and maternal attachment to twins. *J. Obstet. Gynecol. Neonatal Nurs.* 10:120.

Dutton, M.A. May-June 1979. A breast feeding protocol. *J. Obstet. Gynecol. Neonatal Nurs.* 8:151.

Freeman, K. March 1980. A postpartum program that really works . . . . help for new mothers as near as the phone. *Can. Nurse.* 76:40.

Gara, E. January-February 1981. Nursing protocol to improve the effectiveness of the contraceptive diaphragm. *MCN.* 6:41.

Gorrie, T.M. January-February 1979. A postpartum evaluation tool. *J. Obstet. Gynecol. Neonatal Nurs.* 8:41.

Gromada, K. March-April 1981. Maternal-infant attachment: the first step toward individualizing twins. *MCN.* 6:129.

Hames, C.T. September-October 1980. Sexual needs and interest of postpartum couples. *J. Obstet. Gynecol. Neonatal Nurs.* 9:313.

Harris, J.K. March 1980. Self-care is possible after cesarean delivery. *Nurs. Clin. North Am.* 15:191.

Hatcher. R.A., et al. 1982. *Contraceptive Technology 1982–1983,* 11th ed. New York: Irvington Publishers, Inc.

Huxall, L.K. May-June 1980. Update on IUD. *MCN.* 5:186.

Inglis, T. September-October 1980. Postpartum sexuality. *J. Obstet. Gynecol. Neonatal Nurs.* 9:298.

Jenkins, R.L., and Westhus, N.K. March-April 1981. The nurse role in parent-infant bonding: overview, assessment, intervention. *J. Obstet. Gynecol. Neonatal Nurs.* 10:114.

Jimenez, S.L., and Jungman, R.G. September-October 1980. Supplemental information for the family with a multiple pregnancy. *MCN.* 5:320.

Ketter, D.E., and Shelton, B.J. March-April 1983. In-hospital exercises for the postpartal woman. *MCN.* 8(4):120.

Marecki, M.P. July-August 1979. Postpartum follow-up goals and assessment. *J. Obstet. Gynecol. Neonatal Nurs.* 8:214.

Pinckney, C.R. March-April 1981. The bottle baby controversy. *J. Nurs Midwifery.* 26:34.

Riesch, S. July-August 1979. Enhancement of mother-infant social interaction. *J. Obstet. Gynecol. Neonatal Nurs.* 8:242.

Riordan, J., and Countryman, B.A. July-August 1980. Basics of breastfeeding, part I: infant feeding patterns past and present; part II: the anatomy and psychophysiology of lactation. *J. Obstet. Gynecol. Neonatal Nurs.* 9:207.

Riordan, J., and Countryman, B.A. September-October 1980. Basics of breastfeeding, part III: the biological specificity of breast milk; part IV: preparation for breastfeeding and early optimal functioning. *J. Obstet. Gynecol. Neonatal Nurs.* 9:273.

Riordan, J., and Countryman, B.A. November-December 1980. Basics of breastfeeding, part V: self-care for continued breastfeeding, part VI: some breastfeeding problems and solutions. *J. Obstet. Gynecol. Neonatal Nurs.* 9:357.

Riordan, J.M., and Rapp, E.T. March-April 1980. Pleasure and purpose: the sensuousness of breastfeeding. *J. Obstet. Gynecol. Neonatal Nurs.* 9:109.

Schlegel, A.M. May-June 1983. Observations on breastfeeding technique: facts and fallacies. *MCN.* 8(3):204.

Sheehan, F. January-February 1981. Assessing postpartum adjustment: a pilot study. *J. Obstet. Gynecol. Neonatal Nurs.* 10:19.

Strelnick, E.G. July-August 1982. Postpartum care: an opportunity to reinforce breast self-examination. *MCN.* 7(4):249.

Sweeney, S.L., and Davis, F.B. Spring 1979. Transition to parenthood: a group experience. *Maternal-Child Nurs. J.* 8:59.

Tibbetts, E., and Cadwell, K. July-August 1980. Selecting the right breast pump. *MCN.* 5:262.

CHAPTER 13 COMPLICATIONS OF THE POSTPARTAL PERIOD

INTRODUCTION

The postpartal period is regarded by some as rather anticlimatic. The great drama of labor and delivery is completed, and there seems to be little else to do. In reality this is far from true. After even the most uneventful delivery, nursing assessments of mother and baby are essential. The emotional support and teaching a postpartal nurse provides cannot be overemphasized, nor can the nurse's responsibility to carefully monitor the patient's physical status. Complications do sometimes develop during the postpartal period, but their severity may often be ameliorated by early detection and intervention.

This chapter is designed to explore the complications that may arise during the postpartal period. It begins with hemorrhage, the major risk for the childbearing mother. It then goes on to consider other potential complications and ends with disorders of bonding.

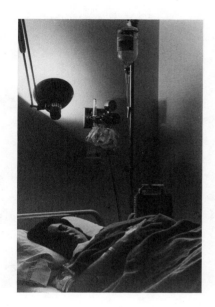

PART I
GENERAL PRINCIPLES AND CONCEPTS

Postpartum Hemorrhage

1. A blood loss of more than _____ mL is classified as postpartum hemorrhage.

2. Postpartum hemorrhage may be classified as early or late. Describe the time of onset and primary cause(s) of each.

   a. Early

   b. Late

3. List five contributing factors that predispose a mother to postpartum hemorrhage.

a.

b.

c.

d.

e.

Joan Burke, a 33-year-old gravida III para III, is admitted to your recovery room following delivery of twin boys. Her labor lasted 2½ hours.

4. Identify two factors that predispose Joan to early postpartum hemorrhage.*

a.

b.

5. During your assessment of Joan, what three findings would indicate possible postpartum hemorrhage?

a.

b.

c.

*These questions are addressed at the end of Part I.

6. What nursing interventions should be initiated for a patient demonstrating signs of postpartum hemorrhage?

Subinvolution

7. Define *subinvolution*.

8. Identify two nursing assessments that would lead you to suspect subinvolution.*

   a.

   b.

9. Identify four interventions that are indicated in the treatment of subinvolution.

   a.

   b.

   c.

   d.

Carrie Spencer begins to complain of severe rectal pain shortly after her vaginal delivery. You note a small area of swelling to the right of her midline episiotomy. Her vital signs are blood pressure 120/88, pulse 80, respiration 20.

10. List three nursing interventions that you should institute at this time.*

    a.

*These questions are addressed at the end of Part I.

   b.

   c.

11. After 30 minutes, Carrie is still experiencing severe rectal pain. You note that the area of swelling has increased in size. Now her vital signs are blood pressure 100/70, pulse 90, respiration 20.

   a. Carrie probably has a _____.*

   b. What pertinent facts should be reported to the physician?

12. Describe the anticipated treatment of a hematoma.

Puerperal Infections

13. How does the Joint Committee on Maternal Welfare define *puerperal morbidity*?

14. Identify four factors that increase a woman's susceptibility to infection during labor and delivery.

   a.

   b.

c.

d.

15. Complete the following chart on puerperal infection:

COMPONENT	LOCALIZED INFECTION (EPISIOTOMY AND/ OR LACERATION)	ENDOMETRITIS	PARAMETRITIS
Tissues involved			
Clinical manifestations			
Interventions			
Complications			

16. Identify criteria that can be used to evaluate the effectiveness of treatment of puerperal infections.*

*These questions are addressed at the end of Part I.

Mastitis

One week after her discharge, Alice, a 23-year-old gravida I para I, who is breast-feeding her infant, develops mastitis.

17. List two factors that contribute to the development of mastitis.

    a.

    b.

18. The most common causative organism of mastitis is _____.

19. Identify four clinical manifestations of mastitis that Alice may exhibit.

    a.

    b.

    c.

    d.

20. What treatment measures would you expect to be instituted for Alice?

21. Compare the various opinions about continuing breast-feeding during an episode of mastitis.

Thromboembolic Disease

22. Define each of the following thromboembolic diseases, describing the clinical manifestations of each:

a. Superficial thrombophlebitis

b. Pelvic thrombosis

c. Deep vein thrombosis

d. Pulmonary embolism

23. Discuss the physiologic changes of pregnancy that increase a woman's susceptibility to blood clot formation during the postpartal period.

24. List two diagnostic tests used to identify thrombophlebitis.

    a.

    b.

25. Identify three interventions that are useful in preventing the development of thrombophlebitis during the postpartal period.

    a.

    b.

    c.

26. Describe the appropriate interventions for a mother with deep vein thrombophlebitis.

27. What medication would you expect a patient with thrombophlebitis to receive initially?

28. Identify three signs of anticoagulant overdose.

    a.

    b.

    c.

29. The antagonist of heparin is _____.

30. What special instructions should be given to a patient receiving Dicumerol?

Puerperal Cystitis

31. List three factors that predispose the postpartal woman to the development of cystitis.

    a.

    b.

    c.

32. Identify four clinical manifestations of cystitis.

   a.

   b.

   c.

   d.

33. Identify appropriate interventions in the treatment of the patient with cystitis.

It is the third postpartal day for Bonnie Sumpter, an 18-year-old primipara. She is single and is keeping her baby. In team conference her nurse expresses concern that she is not bonding appropriately with her infant.

34. Identify four behaviors that might indicate inadequate maternal bonding.

   a.

   b.

   c.

   d.

35. Discuss ways in which the nurse can assist Bonnie in bonding with her infant.

Selected Answers

This section addresses the asterisked questions found in this chapter.

4. Joan is predisposed to early postpartum hemorrhage because of overdistention of the uterus, which is present with a full-term multiple pregnancy and because of her precipitous labor.

8. Two key nursing assessments that would lead you to suspect subinvolution are noting that the uterus is not decreasing in size at the expected rate and prolongation of lochia rubra or return of lochia rubra after the first several days of the postpartal period. Breast-feeding assists in involution, as you know, but you should not rule out the possibility of subinvolution in breast-feeding mothers if these signs exist.

10. Based on the information you were given, you should continue to monitor vital signs every 15 minutes, assess the perineum for any increase in the amount of swelling, and apply an ice pack to the perineum. (Placement of an ice pack is allowed in many institutions without a doctor's order. Application of cold will help decrease swelling caused by trauma to the tissues.)

11. a. Carrie has a hematoma. Were you able to indentify this problem? If not, review the signs and symptoms of hematoma in your textbook.

16. Evaluation criteria would include

 a. signs of wound healing, such as decreased drainage, swelling, or redness of tissues.
 b. normal temperature.
 c. increased tolerance for ambulation.
 d. understanding by the patient of the treatment regimen, self-care, preventive measures, and implications for care of her newborn.

Your evaluation criteria may differ from these but should address some of these aspects.

PART II
SELF-ASSESSMENT GUIDE

The following multiple-choice questions will help you assess your knowledge of the content of this chapter. Select the best answer for each of the questions and then refer to the end of Part II to check your answers.

1. The clinical manifestations of a localized infection of the episiotomy would include

 a. reddened, edematous tissue with yellowish discharge.
 b. reddened, bruised tissue.
 c. approximation of skin edges of the episiotomy.
 d. patient complaints of severe discomfort in the perineum and an oral temperature of 99.8°F (37.7°C).

Marie Walker has recently delivered and states that she has a history of thrombophlebitis. Questions #2 through #6 are related to Marie's condition.

2. Which of the following nursing measures will be most important for Marie in light of her history?

   a. Maintain bed rest.
   b. Encourage Marie to rest in bed with the knee gatch up.
   c. Encourage early ambulation.
   d. Assess vital signs frequently.

3. Marie has developed thrombophlebitis and is receiving heparin intravenously. It will be important to watch her for signs of overdose, which include

   a. hematuria, ecchymosis, and vertigo.
   b. epistaxis, hematuria, and dysuria.
   c. hematuria, ecchymosis, and epistaxis.
   d. dysuria.

4. You know that a drug used to combat problems related to overdoses of heparin is

   a. protamine sulfate.
   b. protamine zinc.
   c. calcium gluconate.
   d. calcium sulfate.

5. As you talk with Marie, she suddenly complains of dyspnea and chest pain. Marie has developed

   a. another thrombophlebitis.
   b. a drug reaction to heparin.
   c. an inflammatory reaction.
   d. pulmonary embolism.

6. A positive Homan's sign is indicated by a complaint of pain in

   a. the leg when the foot is dorsiflexed while the knee is held flat.
   b. the foot when the patient stands.
   c. the leg when the knee is flexed and the foot is extended.
   d. the leg when the knee is held flat and the foot is rotated.

7. Naomi Brookens, a breast-feeding mother, develops mastitis. The clinical manifestations of mastitis include

   a. marked engorgement, high temperature, chills, and pain.
   b. a hard, warm nodular area in the outer quadrant of the breast.
   c. cessation of lactation.
   d. marked engorgement and pain.

8. A neighbor who had a cesarean birth 10 days ago calls to ask your advice. She tells you that she has lochia rubra and is still using eight maternity pads a day. You would suspect which of the following?

   a. Endometritis
   b. Parametritis
   c. Subinvolution
   d. Nothing, because this is a normal course for a cesarean birth

Answers

1. a   5. d
2. c   6. a
3. c   7. a
4. a   8. c

SELECTED BIBLIOGRAPHY

Clarke-Pearson, D.L., and Creasman, W.T. July 1981. Diagnosis of deep venous thrombosis in obstetrics and gynecology by impedance phlebography. *Obstet. Gynecol.* 58:52.

Devore, N.E. July-August 1979. The relationship between previous elective abortions and postpartum depressive reactions. *J. Obstet. Gynecol. Neonatal Nurs.* 8:237.

Eschenbach, D., and Wager, G. December 1980. Puerperal infections. *Clin. Obstet. Gynecol.* 23:1003.

Ezrati, J.B., and Gordon, H. November-December 1979. Puerperal mastitis: causes, prevention, and management. *J. Nurs. Midwifery.* 24:3.

Gibbs, R.S. May 1980 supplement. Clinical risk factors for puerperal infection. *Obstet. Gynecol.* 55:1715.

Gibbs, R.S., et al. November 1980. Endometritis following vaginal delivery. *Obstet. Gynecol.* 56:555.

Nyman, J.E.S. January 1980. Thrombophlebitis in pregnancy. *AJN.* 80:90.

Shy, K.K., and Eschenbach, D.A. September 1979. Fatal perineal cellulitis from an episiotomy site. *Obstet. Gynecol.* 54:292.

Spaulding, L.B., et al. April 1979. The role of ultrasonography in the management of endometritis/salpingitis/peritonitis. *Obstet. Gynecol.* 53:442.

Tentoni, S.C., and High, K.A. July-August 1980. Culturally induced postpartum depression: a theoretical position. *J. Obstet. Gynecol. Neonatal Nurs.* 9:246.

CHAPTER 14 NURSING ASSESSMENT AND CARE OF THE NEONATE

INTRODUCTION

The extrauterine adaptation of the newborn infant is far more complex and exacting than previously recognized. The physiologic changes that occur are at once dramatic and yet subtle, requiring careful and continuous monitoring. Today's neonatal nurse assesses neonatal development, identifies common variations in each newborn, and recognizes abnormalities. The nurse also monitors the neonate's changing status, institutes interventions as needed, and evaluates their effectiveness.

Patient education, a second major area of nursing responsibility, involves helping the family learn to care for its newest member. Inadequate parental understanding of the neonate's needs and requirements may jeopardize its health status and even its existence.

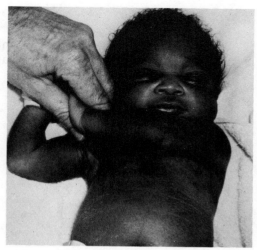

This chapter focuses on the normal physiologic changes that occur in the newborn. It then considers the assessments, early nursing interventions, and health teaching that are required for successful functioning of the parent-infant unit.

PART I
GENERAL PRINCIPLES AND CONCEPTS

1. Describe four factors that are thought to stimulate the newborn to take its first breath.

   a.

   b.

    c.

    d.

2. State four anatomic and physiologic changes that occur in the cardiovascular system during the transition from fetal to neonatal circulation.*

    a.

    b.

    c.

    d.

3. Describe the changes in physiologic functioning that occur in the following systems during the neonatal period:

SYSTEM	NEONATAL PHYSIOLOGIC ADAPTATION
Hepatic	

*These questions are addressed at the end of Part I.

SYSTEM	NEONATAL PHYSIOLOGIC ADAPTATION
Gastrointestinal Digestive enzymes	
Salivary glands	
Cardiac sphincter	
Lower bowel	
Renal Characteristics	
Specific gravity	
Urine output	
Immunologic	

4. List the normal blood values in the newborn for each of the following:

   a. Red blood cells

   b. White blood cells

   c. Hemoglobin

   d. Hematocrit

   e. Bilirubin

   f. Arterial blood gases

5. List the normal values for the following areas of initial assessment of the neonate:

ASSESSMENT AREA	NORMAL VALUES
Temperature	
Pulse	
Respirations	
Blood pressure	
Average weight of white infant in U.S.	
Average weight of nonwhite infant in U.S.	

ASSESSMENT AREA	NORMAL VALUES
Average length of a male	
Average length of a female	
Circumference of the head	
Circumference of the chest	

Newborn Admission

6. The labor and delivery nurse and father arrive in the admission area with Ryan, age 20 minutes. What six essential areas of information should you ascertain from the nurse about Ryan's intranatal and immediate postnatal period? Give your rationale.*

    a.

    b.

    c.

    d.

    e.

    f.

7. List six nursing actions you would perform when admitting a newborn to the nursery.*

    a.

*These questions are addressed at the end of Part I.

b.

c.

d.

e.

f.

8. As part of the initial admission process, a newborn's rectal temperature is taken. What is the reason for determining a newborn's temperature this way?

9. Why are the newborn's hands and feet often cold?

10. Newborns can lose body heat through four mechanisms. Complete the following chart, stating the method of body heat loss and preventive measures that can be taken:

LOSS OF BODY HEAT	PREVENTIVE MEASURES
a.	
b.	
c.	
d.	

11. On Figure 14-1, draw a series of numbered circles to indicate the correct sequence for auscultating a newborn's lungs. Place an X at the point where you should place your stethoscope in order to count the apical pulse.

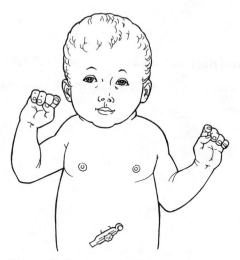

Figure 14-1. Auscultation of newborn's lungs and heart.

12. Draw dotted lines on Figure 14-2 to show where you would measure a newborn's head and chest.

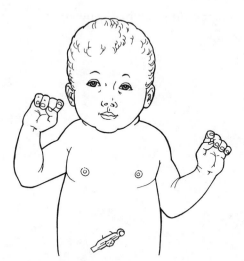

Figure 14-2. Measurement of newborn's head and chest.

13. What might a variation in the proportion of the head-to-chest circumferences indicate?

14. How do you accurately and safely measure the newborn's length?

15. Usual weight loss within the first 3-4 days of life for a full-term newborn is _____%.

16. Why does the newborn commonly exhibit a "physiologic weight loss"?

17. What is the expected difference in average weight between male and female newborn infants?

18. State four factors that influence the weight of a newborn.

    a.

    b.

    c.

    d.

19. Why is a vitamin K medication given prophylactically to newborns?

20. What is the appropriate dosage for administration of vitamin K? _____

21. What is the preferred site for administering intramuscular injections to newborns?

22. Prophylactic eye ointments are instilled in the newborn's eyes in the immediate newborn period to prevent _____, which is caused by _____.

23. List two prophylactic eye ointments that are commonly used.

    a.

    b.

24. For each of the following laboratory values, identify the significance and appropriate nursing interventions:

LABORATORY VALUE	SIGNIFICANCE	NURSING INTERVENTION
Central hematocrit of 68%		
Hemoglobin of 12.5 gm/dL		
Bilirubin of 15 mg/dL		

25. Define *gestational age.*

26. List five physical components that are assessed in determining gestational age by either the Lubchenco or Dubowitz method.

    a.

    b.

c.

d.

e.

27. List four neurologic assessments used in determining gestational age.
    a.

    b.

    c.

    d.

28. What factors might influence the neonate's gestational age score?*

29. Why is it important to determine the gestational age of all newborns?

*These questions are addressed at the end of Part I.

The normal newborn passes through specific periods of reactivity while making the transition to extrauterine life.

30. Complete the following chart:

PERIOD	TIME OF ONSET	NEONATAL CHARACTERISTICS	NURSING INTERVENTION
First period of reactivity			
First period of rest and sleep			
Second period of reactivity			

31. While working in the nursery, you notice that baby Lewis, age 5 hours, has turned blue. Closer inspection reveals a large amount of frothy mucus in his mouth. What immediate nursing interventions would you undertake?*

32. As the newborn nursery nurse, you would complete an initial physical assessment of each newborn. How would you proceed to do this physical assessment?

33. Complete the physical assessment chart on pp. 266-271.

*These questions are addressed at the end of Part I.

ASSESSMENT AREA	NORMAL FINDINGS	COMMON VARIATIONS	DEVIATIONS
Posture At rest			
Awake			
Skin Color			
Texture			
Head Shape			
Sutures			
Fontanelles			

Face

Eyes
Placement

Color and focus

Movement

Conjunctiva

Ears
Appearance

Placement

Nose

ASSESSMENT AREA	NORMAL FINDINGS	COMMON VARIATIONS	DEVIATIONS
Mouth Lips			
Gums			
Palate			
Tongue			
Neck Appearance			
Movement			
Clavicles			

Chest
Shape

Breast

Heart

Characteristics of
pulse

Lungs

Characteristics
of breathing

Cry

ASSESSMENT AREA	NORMAL FINDINGS	COMMON VARIATIONS	DEVIATIONS
Abdomen Shape and size			
Umbilical cord vessels			
Hips			
Extremities Position			
Shape			
Movement			
Color			

Genitalia
Male

Female

Back
General appearance

Spine

Anus
Placement

Patency

34. Discuss the expected level of development in the newborn of the following senses:

SENSE	LEVEL OF DEVELOPMENT
Sight	
Hearing	
Touch	
Taste	
Smell	
Pain	

35. Identify methods that may be used to assess the newborn's vision and hearing.

36. Identify each of the following newborn skin variations, differentiating them by appearance, location, and significance:
    a. Harlequin color change

    b. Erythema neonatorum toxicum

    c. Telangiectatic nevi (stork bites)

    d. Nevus flammeus (port-wine stain)

   e. Mongolian spots

   f. Nevus vasculosis (strawberry mark)

37. Define *molding*.

38. Compare cephalhematoma and caput succedaneum.

CHARACTERISTIC	CAPUT SUCCEDANEUM	CEPHALHEMATOMA
Onset		
Location		
Composition		
Duration		

39. What is the significance of the following variations of the fontanelles?
   a. Bulging

   b. Depressed

40. What position do most newborns usually assume? Why?

41. What motor activity would you expect to see in a newborn that is

    a. Sleeping?

    b. Awake?

42. What changes in the neonate's motor activity would make you suspect neonatal tetany?

43. How is neonatal hypocalcemia treated?

44. Identify four indicators of congenital dislocated hip(s).

    a.

    b.

    c.

    d.

45. The newborn is born with various reflexes. Complete the following chart:

REFLEX	DESCRIPTION	HOW ELICITED	AGE AT DIS-APPEARANCE
Moro			
Tonic neck			
Rooting			
Grasp			
Stepping			
Other			

46. Identify four protective reflexes found in all normal newborns.

a.

b.

c.

d.

47. After completing the physical assessment of a newborn, deviations may be identified. Define each of the following deviations:

a. Hydrocephalus

b. Facial nerve palsy

c. Cleft lip

d. Polydactyly

e. Syndactyly

f. Omphalocele

g. Hypospadias

h. Myelomeningocele

i. Clubfoot

48. On your postpartal unit, you are conducting mother's classes on newborn characteristics. The mothers express concerns about the following common occurrences. How would you respond to each?

a. "Can I hurt him by washing his hair over that soft spot? When will it close?"

b. "All my family's eyes are brown, but her eyes are blue."

c. "Why are there tiny white spots across the bridge of her nose and on her chin?"

d. "Are my baby's eyes alright? There are bright red marks on the white part of his eyes."

e. "He has white patches in his mouth. Is that milk? How can you determine the cause?"

f. "My son's breasts are so swollen. Will the swelling go down?"

g. "My baby is still losing weight. When will it stop?"

h. "When I changed her diaper, there was blood on it."

i. "Are her feet clubbed? They turn in."

j. List other questions you have been asked by mothers and your response to them.

49. Mrs. Smith, a gravida III para III breech delivery, unwraps her son's blanket for the first time to change his diaper. She suddenly puts on her call light. As you enter her room, she exclaims, "Look at his legs! They are up to his stomach and his buttock is bruised." How would you respond to her concern?

Daily Newborn Nursing Assessments

50. You are assigned to the regular newborn nursery. List seven daily assessments that should be made of each newborn.*

a.

b.

c.

d.

e.

*These questions are addressed at the end of Part I.

f.

g.

51. Define *physiologic jaundice*.

52. How would you explain physiologic jaundice to a new mother?

53. Why is the time of onset of jaundice important?

54. Ryan is 12 hours old, and he voids as you begin to change his diaper. What observations should you make about his voiding?

55. You also note that Ryan's wet diaper has a pinkish rust color in the voided area. What is the cause of this?

56. What might a failure to void within the first 24 hours of life indicate?

57. You would expect Ryan to have his first stool within _____ hours after birth.

58. Describe the typical appearance of a neonate's first stool.

59. If Ryan doesn't pass his first stool within the appropriate time, what might this indicate?

60. When do transitional stools occur, and what are their characteristics?

61. Complete the following chart comparing the stools of breast-fed and formula-fed infants:

CHARACTERISTIC OF STOOLS	BREAST-FED	FORMULA-FED
Frequency		
Color		
Consistency		
Odor		

62. Ryan is given sterile water for his first feeding. Why are most newborns given sterile water first?

63. What nursing interventions would you carry out to evaluate the adequacy of Ryan's fluid and nutritional intake while being breast-fed?*

*These questions are addressed at the end of Part I.

64. The average daily caloric requirement for a full-term newborn is _____cal/kg, or _____cal/lb, and the daily fluid requirement is _____ml/kg.

65. Christy is a 2-day-old bottle-fed infant. Her mother is concerned because "she only takes 1½ oz at each feeding." What would be your response?

66. Christy is discharged at 3 days of age. She should have a daily intake of approximately _____oz and, by the time she is 1 month old, _____oz.

67. Christy's mother is concerned about the care of Christy's umbilical cord at home.

    a. What information would you give her about the expected changes in the umbilical cord from birth until the cord separates from the infant?

    b. What information about daily assessments and care of the cord should you give Christy's mother?

    c. She asks, "When can I give Christy a bath?" How would you respond?

68. Prior to discharge, Ryan is circumcised.

    a. What are your nursing responsibilities during and following the circumcision?

    b. What home-care instructions would you provide?

69. Michael, a 3-day-old uncircumcised newborn, is ready for discharge. What instructions should you give his mother about penile care?

70. What type of immunity does the newborn receive from its mother?

71. List the nursing measures that are necessary to protect the newborn from infection in the hospital.

72. As newborn Michael is being readied for discharge, his mother mentions that her 3-year-old has just come home from preschool with measles.

    a. What information must you elicit from her in order to determine the significance for Michael?

b. What health teaching is indicated for Michael's mother?

73. You are to present a newborn discharge teaching program.

a. List the essential components of this teaching program.*

b. How might you evaluate the effectiveness of your teaching?

74. Taking a new baby home brings changes within a family.

a. What changes in lifestyle might they anticipate?

*These questions are addressed at the end of Part I.

b. What guidance can you give to help ease the baby into the family?

Selected Answers

This section addresses the asterisked questions found in this chapter.

2. The newborn's cardiovascular system accomplishes the following anatomic and physiologic alterations during the transition from fetal to neonatal circulation:
   a. Increase in aortic pressure and decrease in venous pressure as a result of loss of the placenta
   b. Increased systemic pressure and decreased pulmonary artery pressure due to decreased pulmonary circulatory resistance and vasodilatation
   c. Closure of the ductus venosus and foramen ovale
   d. Closure of the ductus arteriosis, which increases blood flow in the pulmonary vascular tree

   If you have identified these alterations, you have increased your understanding of what is necessary for the neonate to function as a new, independent individual.

6. As the admitting nursery nurse, you should ascertain the following essential areas of information from the labor and delivery nurse:

   a. Problems occurring during labor and delivery, such as signs of fetal distress or maternal problems (abruptio placentae, preeclampsia, and prolapse of the cord, all of which compromise the fetus in utero)
   b. Medications given to the mother during labor or given to the neonate in the immediate postdelivery period.
   c. The baby's Apgar scores
   d. Resuscitative measures administered to the newborn
   e. Elimination during the postdelivery period (did the neonate void or pass meconium in the delivery room?)
   f. General condition and activity level

   If you identified these areas, you have a basis for identifying significant potential problems for the neonate. These areas of information provide a data base from which to make continued careful and significant observations during the transition period.

7. Nursing actions that you would perform when admitting a neonate to the nursery include

   a. noting vital signs (including blood pressure in some agencies)
   b. measuring weight
   c. measuring length
   d. taking head and chest measurements
   e. scoring for gestational age
   f. administering prophylactic medications

   In addition, many institutions do a general head-to-toe admission physical assessment and blood work (Hct and Dextrostix). Other institutions also do stomach aspirations, but this procedure is controversial and shouldn't be done until the neonate is stablized because it can cause bradycardia and apnea.

28. Factors that can influence a neonate's gestational age scores are

   a. medications (especially on the assessment of the neurologic components).
   b. anoxia or hypoxia, which can result in decreased muscle tone and reflex determinations.
   c. timing of the scoring. For example, if sole creases are evaluated after 12 hours, the natural drying of the soles increases what appears to be sole creases; or if the labor and delivery nurse thoroughly removes the vernix before the gestational score is determined, the score will be inaccurate.
   d. variations in the usual physical characteristics because of intrauterine conditions. For example, the infant of a diabetic mother and the premature large-for-gestational-age infant both have more breast tissue (increased subcutaneous tissue) than an infant of true gestational maturation.
   e. difficult delivery, which may make determination of skull firmness difficult.

31. You would immediately aspirate the mouth and nasal pharynx with a bulb syringe, holding the neonate with its head down and neck extended to facilitate drainage as you aspirate the mucus.
   If you also recognize that there is an increase in mucus production during the second period of reactivity, you are well on your way to being alert and prepared to intervene in this very real problem.

50. Daily neonatal assessments should include

   a. vital signs.
   b. weight.
   c. overall color.
   d. stool pattern.
   e. voiding pattern.
   f. caloric and fluid intake.
   g. cord care.

63. The adequacy of the fluid and caloric intake of a breast-fed infant is determined by weighing him or her before and after nursing and by observing the quantity of urine and feces and their patterns of elimination.

73. a. Essential components of a newborn discharge teaching program would include the following:

   bathing (skin, scalp, and nail care)
   eye and ear care
   nasal suctioning (use of a bulb syringe)
   cord care
   circumcision care or care of the uncircumcised male infant
   care of female genitalia
   diapering
   positioning and handling
   establishing a feeding schedule versus feeding on demand
   burping
   pumping the breasts and supplemental feedings for breast-fed infants
   formula preparation
   introduction to solids (what, when, why)
   providing vitamin supplements
   stooling and voiding patterns
   sleep patterns
   clothing
   neonatal behavioral changes after discharge
   observation for signs of illness
   use of thermometer
   testing for phenylketonuria
   pediatric followup

PART II
SELF-ASSESSMENT GUIDE

The following multiple-choice questions will help assess your knowledge of the content of this chapter. Select the best answer for each of the questions then refer to the end of Part II to check your answers.

1. The normal breathing pattern for a full-term infant is predominately

   a. diaphragmatic with chest lag.
   b. shallow and irregular respirations.
   c. chest breathing with nasal flaring.
   d. abdominal with synchronous chest movements.

2. The average apical pulse range of a full-term quiet, awake newborn is

   a. 80–100 beats per minute
   b. 100–120 beats per minute
   c. 120–140 beats per minute
   d. 150–180 beats per minute

3. Robert Scott is brought to the nursery by his father and the labor and delivery nurse. He weighs 8 lb and is 21 inches long. You would tell his father that he is

   a. above the average weight and above the average length.
   b. the average weight and above the average length.
   c. the average weight and length.
   d. below the average weight and below the average length.

4. Robert's blood values at 1 day of age are as follows. Which is *not* within normal limits?

   a. Hemoglobin 17.2 gm/dL
   b. Platelets 250,000/mm³
   c. Blood glucose 30 mg/dL
   d. White blood cells 15,000/mm³

5. At 3 days of age, Robert is circumcised. Which of the following rationales governs his post-circumcision care?

   a. Bleeding from the operative site may occur within the first 12 hours after the circumcision.
   b. The wound must be kept clean to prevent contamination of the incision.
   c. Vaseline acts as a lubricant to help prevent diaper irritation.
   d. All of the above.

6. Which of the following assessments would *not* require immediate notification of the physician?

   a. Failure to pass meconium during the first 24 hours of life
   b. Failure to void during the first 24 hours of life
   c. Inability to pass a rectal thermometer more than ⅛ inch into the rectum
   d. Pink or rusty-colored stains on a diaper with voiding

7. Vitamin K is administered in the immediate neonatal period because

   a. hemolysis of the fetal red blood cells increases coagulation problems.
   b. newborns are susceptible to avitaminosis.
   c. newborns lack intestinal bacteria with which to synthesize vitamin K.
   d. a newborn's liver is incapable of producing sufficient vitamin K to deal with transient neonatal coagulation problems.

8. While making rounds in the nursery, you see a 6-hour-old newborn gagging and turning bluish. You would first

   a. alert the physician.
   b. aspirate the oral and nasal pharynx.
   c. give oxygen by positive pressure.
   d. lower the infant's head and stimulate crying.

9. A 3-day-old newborn would be expected to have a fluid intake per feeding of

   a. ½-1 oz
   b. 1½-2 oz
   c. 2-3 oz
   d. 3-5 oz

10. Newborns often regurgitate easily after feedings because

   a. their stomach is small and easily overfills.
   b. control of their cardiac sphincter is immature.
   c. control of their pyloric sphincter is immature.
   d. peristalsis is reversed in their esophagus.

Answers

1. d	6. d
2. c	7. c
3. c	8. b
4. c	9. c
5. d	10. b

SELECTED BIBLIOGRAPHY

Buckner, E.B. January-February 1983. Use of Brazetlon neonatal behavioral assessment in planning care for parents and newborns. *JOGN Nurs.* 12:26.

Capobianco, J.A. May 1980. How to safeguard the infant against life-threatening heat loss. *Nurs 80.* 10:64.

Davis, V. November-December 1980. The structure and function of brown adipose tissue in the neonate. *J. Obstet. Gynecol. Neonatal Nurs.* 9:368.

Deters, G.E. July-August 1980. Circadian rhythm phenomenon. *MCN.* 5:249.

Dunn, D.M., and White, D.G. June 1981. Interactions of mothers with their newborns in the first half-hour of life. *J. Advanced Nurs.* 6:271.

Haddock, N. March-April 1980. Blood pressure monitoring in neonates. *MCN.* 5:131.

Hill, S.T., and Shronk, L.K. September-October 1979. The effect of early parent-infant contact on newborn body temperature. *J. Obstet. Gynecol. Neonatal Nurs.* 8:287.

Lubchenco, L.O. December 1980. Routine neonatal circumcision: a surgical anachronism. *Clin. Obstet. Gynecol.* 23:1135.

Markesberry, B.A. 1979. Watching baby's diet: a professional and parent guide. *Am. J. Mat. Child Nurs.* 4:177.

Moss, J., and Solomons, H.C. Fall 1979. Swaddling then, there and now: historical, anthropological and current practices. *Maternal-Child Nurs. J.* 8:137.

Osborn, L.M., et al. March 1981. Hygiene care in uncircumcised infants. *Pediatrics.* 67:365.

Sholder, D.A. March-April 1981. Portrait of a newborn. *J. Obstet. Gynecol. Neonatal Nurs.* 10:98.

Snyder, C., et al. November-December 1979. New findings about mothers' antenatal expectations and their relationship to infant development. *MCN.* 4:354.

Sullivan, R., et al. January-February 1979. Determining a newborn's gestational age. *MCN.* 4:38.

Taylor, L.S. May-June 1981. Newborn feeding behaviors and attaching. *MCN.* 6:201.

White, P.L., et al. May 1980. Comparative accuracy of recent abbreviated methods of gestational age determination. *Clin. Pediatr.* 19:319.

Zepeda, M. November-December 1982. Selected maternal-infant care practices of Spanish speaking women. *JOGN Nurs.* 11:371.

CHAPTER 15 *NURSING ASSESSMENT AND CARE OF THE HIGH-RISK NEONATE*

INTRODUCTION

The majority of pregnancies end with the delivery of a healthy term infant who flourishes with appropriate parental care and support. However, some infants develop serious problems during their early hours and days of life. These infants are classified as "high risk." In many instances the maternal or fetal factors that increase risk can be predicted during the antepartal period. In other cases the infant's high-risk status results from insults or complications that occur during labor and delivery. In both instances appropriate interventions can significantly improve the baby's outlook.

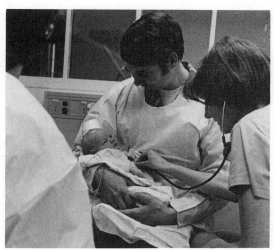

This chapter first considers the factors that contribute to the development of a high-risk infant and the commonly used methods of assessing an infant's status. It then focuses on many of the problems that may afflict high-risk infants, with emphasis on nursing assessments and interventions and, finally, on evaluation of the effectiveness of care.

PART I
GENERAL PRINCIPLES AND CONCEPTS

1. Define the following terms used to identify infants at risk:

    a. Appropriate for gestational age (AGA)

    b. Preterm

    c. Low birthweight

d. Small for gestational age (SGA)

e. Postterm

f. Large for gestational age (LGA)

2. Identify six maternal factors that may contribute to the birth of a high-risk infant.

a.

b.

c.

d.

e.

f.

3. Determination of gestational age is critical in anticipating potential problems. List four potential problems related to each of the following groups of high-risk infants:

a. Preterm

b. SGA

c. LGA

d. Postterm

Preterm Infant

4. List four causes of prematurity.

   a.

   b.

   c.

   d.

5. State two criteria used to classify a newborn as preterm.*

   a.

   b.

6. Describe six physical characteristics you would expect to find in an AGA 35-week gestational age newborn.

   a.

   b.

*These questions are addressed at the end of Part I.

c.

d.

e.

f.

7. You have just received a call from the delivery room that a preterm infant has been born. What preparations and equipment should you get ready in order to receive this infant?*

8. A preterm infant arrives in the nursery. What three initial assessments should you make?*

a.

b.

c.

*These questions are addressed at the end of Part I.

9. The physical characteristics and immaturity of the preterm infant's body systems cause them to exhibit a number of physiologic problems. For each of the following problems, identify the cause and the appropriate nursing interventions:

PHYSIOLOGIC PROBLEM	CAUSE	NURSING INTERVENTIONS
Temperature instability		
Respiratory distress		
Susceptibility to infection		
Adequate caloric and fluid intake		
Hypocalcemia		
Hypoglycemia		

Premature infants are susceptible to temperature instability and should be placed in a regulated environment.

10. Define *neutral thermal environment*.

11. Why is it desirable to maintain a neutral thermal environment for the preterm infant?

12. In what range should the preterm infant's skin temperature be maintained?

If the preterm infant's thermal environment is not maintained, cold stress can occur.

13. Define *cold stress.*

14. What four metabolic changes and resultant problems may occur in the preterm infant as a result of cold stress?*

   a.

   b.

   c.

   d.

15. Describe the nursing interventions that you would institute to prevent or minimize hypothermia/cold stress.

*These questions are addressed at the end of Part I.

Respiratory Distress Syndrome

Tricia, a 3½ lb (1587 g) neonate with a gestational age of 34 weeks, was born at 10:30 PM. Her Apgar score at 1 minute was 3, necessitating resuscitation via intubation and oxygen administration. On admission to the high-risk nursery, her vital signs are pulse 150, respirations 50, and temperature of 96.2°F (35.7°C) (rectal). She is placed in a radiant heat warmer, and an umbilical artery catheter is inserted for intravenous infusion.

16. You are to assess Tricia for signs of respiratory distress. List six signs indicative of developing respiratory distress.*

    a.

    b.

    c.

    d.

    e.

    f.

17. What information does a Silverman-Anderson score provide?

18. What three factors may predispose Tricia to develop respiratory distress syndrome?*

    a.

*These questions are addressed at the end of Part I.

b.

c.

19. Define *respiratory distress syndrome* (hyaline membrane disease).

20. Briefly describe the pathologic sequence involved in respiratory distress syndrome.

21. It is now 2 AM, and Tricia is showing signs of respiratory distress syndrome. She is placed in an oxygen hood with a warmed, humidified oxygen concentration of 70%. What is the rationale for administering warmed and humidified oxygen?

22. Tricia's respirations are now 65 per minute; she has an apical pulse of 152-176 beats per minute; and her arterial blood gases show a pH of 7.3, PO_2 of 55 mm Hg., and PCO_2 of 60 mm Hg.

    a. What are your nursing responsibilities during oxygen administration?*

*These questions are addressed at the end of Part I.

b. How would you evaluate the effectiveness of Tricia's oxygen therapy?

23. Oxygen administration to the premature infant can lead to complications. Briefly discuss the pathology and nursing management of the following:

COMPLICATION	PATHOLOGY	NURSING INTERVENTIONS
Retrolental fibroplasia		
Bronchopulmonary dysplasia		

Tricia is initially maintained on intravenous fluids via umbilical catheter. When her respiratory status improves, she is placed on a half-strength premature formula via gavage feedings every 2 hours.

24. Why is gavage feeding initiated before nipple feedings?

25. List three methods of assessing proper placement of a gavage tube prior to feedings.

a.

b.

c.

298

26. What nursing assessments would you make to determine the following?*

    a. Tricia's tolerance of gavage feedings

    b. Tricia's readiness for nipple feeding

27. What are Tricia's caloric and fluid requirements per kilogram per day?

28. Tricia's mother arrives at the special-care nursery when Tricia is 3 hours old. Describe the information and support you should give Tricia's mother.

    a. Prior to entering the nursery

    b. During her visit with Tricia

29. Why is it advised that parents have early contact with and involvement in their preterm infant's care?

30. As you talk with Tricia's mother, she expresses concern about the physical and mental development of her baby. Based on your knowledge of the growth and development of a preterm infant, how would you respond about the following areas?

    a. Physical development for the first year

*These questions are addressed at the end of Part I.

b. Mental development

c. Emotional and social behavior

31. What criteria will be used to determine Tricia's readiness for discharge to her parents?

32. What observations would you make in assessing Tricia's parents' readiness to take Tricia home?

33. Followup care of preterm infants is often undertaken by the public health nurse. What information should you supply the public health nurse to facilitate Tricia's transition to home care?

SGA Infants

34. List four maternal causes for an SGA infant.

    a.

    b.

    c.

    d.

35. What physical findings would you expect when scoring the gestational age of an SGA infant?*

36. Describe the potential long-term implications for an SGA infant.

Postterm Infants

37. List three obstetric indications of a postterm pregnancy.*

     a.

     b.

     c.

38. Describe the clinical picture of a postterm infant.

39. Describe the potential long-term implications for a postterm infant.

*These questions are addressed at the end of Part I.

Neonatal Jaundice

40. Briefly describe the process of bilirubin conjugation.

41. List three factors that influence the rate and amount of bilirubin conjugation.*

   a.

   b.

   c.

42. State three situations that alter the neonate's ability to conjugate bilirubin.*

   a.

   b.

   c.

43. Compare, in the following chart, physiologic and pathologic jaundice:

CHARACTERISTIC	PHYSIOLOGIC JAUNDICE	PATHOLOGIC JAUNDICE
Cause		
Bilirubin level in premature infant		

*These questions are addressed at the end of Part I.

CHARACTERISTIC	PHYSIOLOGIC JAUNDICE	PATHOLOGIC JAUNDICE
Bilirubin level in full-term infant		
Time of onset		
Effect on infant		

44. Define the following terms asociated with neonatal pathologic jaundice.

   a. Hyperbilirubinemia

   b. Kernicterus

   c. Erythroblastosis fetalis

45. What factors might influence your assessment of the neonate's developing jaundice?*

Hemolytic Disease of the Newborn

Alice, a 7 lb 2 oz infant, is 14 hours old and showing signs of jaundice. She is diagnosed as having hemolytic disease of the newborn.

46. What are two possible causes of hemolytic disease of the newborn?

   a.

   b.

*These questions are addressed at the end of Part I.

47. What maternal and paternal factors might have increased Alice's risk of developing this disease?

    a. Maternal

    b. Paternal

48. Briefly describe the physiologic response of an Rh positive woman to an Rh negative fetus.

49. Identify the tests that might be performed during the prenatal period when an Rh incompatibility is suspected.

50. List three maternal and neonatal laboratory tests used to confirm a diagnosis of hemolytic disease of the newborn.

    a.

    b.

    c.

51. Describe the pathologic changes that occur in a newborn with erythroblastosis fetalis.

52. Complete the following chart of therapies used in the treatment of hemolytic disease:

THERAPY	INDICATIONS FOR USE	ACTION
Intrauterine exchange transfusion		
Neonatal exchange transfusion		
Phototherapy		

53. What are your nursing responsibilities

    a. during a neonatal exchange transfusion?

    b. following a neonatal exchange transfusion?

54. Calcium gluconate is administered for each replacement of 100 mL of blood. Why is this done?

55. What are your nursing responsibilities while a newborn is under phototherapy lights?

56. The most severe form of erythroblastosis fetalis is hydrops fetalis. Describe the pathology of this condition.

57. Describe the clinical picture in hydrops fetalis.

58. List three situations in which an Rh negative woman should be given RhoGAM (include the rationale).

   a.

   b.

   c.

Infant of a Diabetic Mother

59. Richard is a 36 weeks' gestation newborn, weighing 9 lb 12 oz. His admitting nursery information indicates that his mother is a class C diabetic. What physical characteristics would you expect him to have?

60. Identify the cause for Richard's excessive weight.

61. What laboratory test should be carried out on Richard and when?

62. You would anticipate Richard's blood glucose at birth to be _____.

63. Richard will show beginning signs of hypoglycemia _____ hours after delivery.

64. Hypoglycemia occurs when blood glucose levels fall below _____ mg/dL.

65. What signs of developing hypoglycemia would you observe in Richard?

66. Identify the interventions you would carry out relative to the assessment and treatment of hypoglycemia.

67. Richard is susceptible to the following complications. State the cause and treatment of each.

COMPLICATION	CAUSE	TREATMENT
Hyperbilirubinemia		
Hypocalcemia		
Respiratory distress		
Birth trauma		

Neonatal Infections

68. Jane is an 8 lb baby girl whose mother had active syphilis. List eight symptoms of congenital syphilis you might expect to see during Jane's neonatal period.

   a.

   b.

   c.

   d.

   e.

   f.

   g.

   h.

69. Serologic dilution tests on an infant, based on detection of _____, are usually diagnostically accurate between _____ and _____ months of age.

70. Describe five nursing measures you would include in your care of a baby like Jane.*

   a.

   b.

   c.

d.

e.

71. You are taking care of Andy, who is 2 days old, and note that he is increasingly lethargic and refuses to eat. He is diagnosed as having sepsis neonatorum. List four factors that increase the newborn's susceptibility to infections.

    a.

    b.

    c.

    d.

72. Identify three bacterial organisms that may cause sepsis neonatorum.

    a.

    b.

    c.

73. List five other symptoms that Andy may exhibit as manifestations of sepsis neonatorum.

    a.

    b.

    c.

d.

e.

74. Identify four diagnostic tests that might be done in a septic workup.*

    a.

    b.

    c.

    d.

75. What are your nursing responsibilities while caring for a septic newborn (include your rationale)?

Drug-Addicted Infants

76. Claire, a 2-day-old, 2000 g neonate, is observed to be going through withdrawal. Her 18-year-old mother was addicted to heroin during the pregnancy. List six symptoms of withdrawal you may observe in Claire.

    a.

    b.

    c.

*These questions are addressed at the end of Part I.

d.

e.

f.

77. Describe five nursing interventions that you may implement to help Claire through the withdrawal period.
    a.

    b.

    c.

    d.

    e.

Selected Answers

This section addresses the asterisked questions found in this chapter.

5. Historically, the classification criterion for preterm newborns was primarily weight only (weight less than 2500 g). By itself, weight may prove inaccurate, especially in light of our new knowledge of SGA infants. The most current and accurate criterion is gestational age scoring, which assesses physical and neurologic maturation. Another criterion is determination of gestation by dates of the last menstrual period, prematurity being gestation of less than 37 completed weeks.

7. Basic preparations and equipment necessary for receiving a preterm newborn should include a method for temperature stabilization (isolette or open bed warmer), a method for ventilatory support: oxygen, appropriate size intubation tubes and airways, and suction equipment. In addition, if appropriate for your nursery, you should provide an alternative method for supplying intravenous fluids and for monitoring blood gases (other than through the scalp veins), such as umbilical catheters. In emergency situations, a #5 feeding tube may be placed in the umbilical artery or vein. The availability of ventilatory support such as a respirator is ideal.

   If you have identified the equipment necessary to provide for adequate oxygenation and temperature stabilization, you are prepared to meet the preterm infant's two most crucial initial needs.

8. The three initial assessments you should make on the arrival of a preterm newborn in the nursery are: observation of signs of respiratory distress, core temperature determination to assess whether hypothermia or cold stress will complicate this infant's course, and gestational age determination to identify other potential problems. You may have identified other areas, but these are the essential ones. Refer to your textbook if you had any difficulty identifying the initial needs of the preterm newborn.

14. The metabolic effects of cold stress include: competition for albumin binding sites by increased nonesterified fatty acids causing increased free circulating bilirubin; increased incidence of hypoglycemia resulting from glucose being used for thermogenesis; pulmonary vaso-constriction in response to the release of norepinephrine; and increase in oxygen consumption and metabolic acidosis as the body burns brown fat deposits. If you were successful in identifying these metabolic changes, you will also be aware that these changes may create serious life-threatening problems for the premature infant.

16. Six signs of respiratory distress are the following: tachypnea, inspiratory retractions, expiratory grunting, nasal flaring, cyanosis, and periods of apnea. Other signs you might look for after these six are lung rales or rhonchi, edema, and chin tug.

18. Tricia's history of preterm delivery, a low Apgar score (hypoxic insult), and a low core temperature (cold stress) all are contributing factors to her development of respiratory distress syndrome.

22. a. Nursing responsibilities during oxygen administration include ensuring that the infant's head is under the oxygen hood and that respiratory passages are not obstructed; ensuring that the tubing is connected and free of moisture buildup; seeing that ambient oxygen concentrations are being monitored by oxygen sensors; and ensuring that oxygen delivery devices are calibrated periodically.

26. a. Nursing assessments of Tricia's tolerance of gavage feedings would include observing for any degree of abdominal distention during or after the feeding; a formula residual of less than 1 ml prior to the next feeding; lack of regurgitation; and no apnea, bradycardia, cyanosis, or color changes. A program of alternate gavage and nipple feeding is recommended to decrease the possibility of fatigue during feeding.
    b. Active sucking motions during and between feedings might indicate the preterm infant's readiness for nipple feeding. You would expect the preterm infant who could tolerate nipple feedings to have a weak grasp of the nipple but a strong suck and to show satiety and relief of oral tension as she feeds.

35. Any infant who at birth is at or below the tenth percentile on intrauterine growth charts should be suspected of being small for gestational age. If growth retardation is the result of an acute episode of placental insufficiency, observe the infant for loss of subcutaneous fat and muscle mass, a wide-eyed face, loss of vernix prior to full term, dry and desquamated skin, and the presence of a meconium-stained cord, skin, and nails in a full-term or preterm infant. By your identification of a possible SGA infant, you can be instrumental in meeting his immediate special needs and in reducing the possible long-term sequelae.

37. Obstetric situations that would lead you to suspect a postterm pregnancy include the following: oligohydramnios, weight loss of 3 lb or more per week in the last weeks of pregnancy, meconium-stained amniotic fluid in a full-term infant, palpation of a hard fetal head, high fetal head arrest, and prolonged labor due to uterine inertia, or CPD. Women of high parity (gravida IV or more), primigravidas, and women whose preceding pregnancy was postterm are also more prone to go beyond term in their present pregnancy.

41. The three most prominent factors influencing the rate and amount of bilirubin conjugation are the following: rate of red blood cell hemolysis, degree of liver maturity, and number of available albumin binding sites. In addition, you might remember that even after the bilirubin is conjugated, it can be unconjugated via the "enterohepatic circulation" and thus cause a delay in clearing the bilirubin from the circulatory system. Also, fetal red blood cells have a shorter half-life than adult cells, which increases the rate of hemolysis.

42. Situations that alter the neonate's ability to conjugate bilirubin include the following: bacterial and viral infections; competition for albumin binding sites by drugs, particularly sulfa drugs and salicylates and nonesterified fatty acids; neonatal asphyxia which decreases the binding affinity of bilirubin to albumin; and the many causes of increased red blood cell hemolysis, such as cephalhematoma.

45. Your assessment of developing jaundice may be affected by fluorescent nursery lights with pink tints which mask jaundice; by blue walls and blue blankets; and by the basic pigmentation of the gumline in ethnic people of color.

70. In caring for a neonate with congenital syphilis, your nursing care should include the following, at least initially: isolating the infant, monitoring intake and output, swaddling the neonate for comfort, covering the neonate's hands to prevent scratching, and administering penicillin as the physician orders. Support and education of the parents are also essential in fostering a positive future environment for this neonate.

74. Diagnostic tests that might be done as part of a septic workup are primarily blood, spinal, nasopharyngeal, and urine cultures. If any lesions or reddened areas are noted, cultures from these areas should also be obtained. A complete blood count, chest x-ray, serology, and Gram stains of cerebrospinal fluid, urine, and umbilicus may also be required. Depending on the suspected cause of the sepsis, other tests may include x-rays of various portions of the body, serum IgM level determinations, and stomach aspirations.

PART II
SELF-ASSESSMENT GUIDE

The following multiple-choice questions will help you assess your knowledge of the content of this chapter. Select the best answer for each of the questions and then refer to the end of Part II to check your answers.

1. Which of the following characteristics is indicative of a preterm newborn of 34 weeks' gestation?

    a. The upper two-thirds of the pinna curves inward.
    b. The scalp hair is silky and in silky strands.
    c. The skin is covered with lanugo except for the face.
    d. The sole creases cover the anterior two-thirds of the foot.

On April 18 at 1:45 PM, a 35-week, 1580 g male infant named John was delivered to a 20-year-old primigravida. Questions 2 through 6 relate to this situation.

2. Immediate assessment of John by the nursery nurse would include all of the following *except*

    a. cardiac function.
    b. congenital abnormalities.
    c. respiratory function.
    d. urinary function.

3. John is beginning to show signs of respiratory distress. Determine the priority for the following nursing interventions:

    1. Notify the physician.
    2. If cyanosis occurs, provide oxygen.
    3. Record time, symptoms, degree of symptoms, and whether oxygen relieved the symptoms of respiratory distress.
    4. Apply monitoring electrodes.
    5. Maintain a patent airway.

    a. 2, 1, 5, 4, and 3
    b. 5, 1, 2, 3, and 4
    c. 4, 2, 5, 1, and 3
    d. 5, 2, 1, 4, and 3

4. John's oxygen concentration is carefully regulated, based on his PO_2 and PCO_2 levels, because high blood levels of oxygen

   a. may produce hyperbilirubinemia.
   b. may cause retinal spasms, leading to the development of retrolental fibroplasia.
   c. cause peripheral circulatory collapse.
   d. cause cardiac shunt closures, although the latter are not permanent.

5. John has demonstrated nasal flaring, intercostal retractions, expiratory grunting, and slight cyanosis. An umbilical catheter is inserted with an intravenous infusion of 5% dextrose and water. John should also be placed in

   a. an incubator with heat control.
   b. an incubator with heat, oxygen controls, and humidity.
   c. an open bed warmer with his head slightly elevated under an oxygen hood.
   d. an open bed warmer with his head slightly elevated.

6. John's parents are very anxious when they see him with all the special equipment around him. Your best response to facilitate parent-infant interaction would be to

   a. assure them that they are fortunate to have John in a special-care nursery.
   b. explain the equipment in simple terms, have them wash their hands, and provide an opportunity for them to touch John.
   c. explain the equipment simply and discuss the viability and continued existence of John.
   d. have them wash their hands so they can touch John.

7. The neonate can contract congential syphilis from his mother

   a. at birth.
   b. during the fifth month of pregnancy.
   c. during the second month of pregnancy.
   d. during the seventh month of pregnancy.

8. Infants of diabetic mothers are at high risk for all of the following problems *except*

   a. congenital heart defects.
   b. hypocalcemia.
   c. hypoglycemia.
   d. erythroblastosis fetalis.

9. Your assessment of a newborn experiencing hypoglycemia would include all of the following *except*

   a. apathy and poor muscle tone.
   b. an increase in the respiratory rate.
   c. a soft, weak cry.
   d. twitching or jitteriness.

10. The nursing management of a heroin-addicted newborn experiencing withdrawal includes

   a. administration of methadone and frequent assessment of vital signs.
   b. frequent assessment of vital signs and wrapping the infant snugly in a blanket.
   c. meticulous skin and perineal care and frequent tactile stimulation.
   d. minimal tactile stimulation and the provision of loose, nonrestrictive clothing.

Mrs. Carla Steffens at 38 weeks' gestation, is concerned that her baby may be born with hemolytic anemia of the newborn. Questions 11 through 15 relate to this situation.